# Concise Notes in Oncology for MRCP and MRCS

## Third Edition

**Kefah Mokbel** MB, BS (Lon), FRCS (Eng), MS (Lon), FRCS (Gen)

*Consultant Surgeon with a Specialist Interest in Breast and Endocrine Surgery, St George's Hospital, London Professor at Brunel Institute of Cancer Genetics and Pharmacogenomics (UK)*

Radcliffe Publishing

Oxford ● Seattle

D1585747

**Radcliffe Publishing Ltd**
18 Marcham Road
Abingdon
Oxon OX14 1AA
United Kingdom

**www.radcliffe-oxford.com**
Electronic catalogue and worldwide online ordering facility.

---

First edition 1999 (published by LibraPharm Ltd)
Second edition 2001 (published by LibraPharm Ltd)

British Library Cataloguing in Publication Data

A catalogue record for this book is available from the British Library.

ISBN 1 85775 757 2

Typeset by Advance Typesetting Ltd, Oxford
Printed and bound by TJ International Ltd, Padstow, Cornwall

# Contents

# Preface to the third edition

This book has two objectives. It is intended to provide an accurate, concise source of information on medical and surgical oncology and to serve as a platform on which to build new information generated by the multitude of scientific and clinical disciplines that continuously contribute to improving our understanding of cancer and its management.

Each cancer is presented in an organised format that includes information about epidemiology, aetiology, pathology, clinical features, investigations, treatment and prognosis.

However, the approach adopted in this book is limited by the amount of detail that can be provided, and it makes no allowances for controversial opinions.

This publication will be valuable to undergraduate medical students preparing for final examinations, postgraduate doctors preparing for the MRCP and MRCS examinations, general practitioners, oncology nurses and basic science researchers in the field of oncology. It will also serve as a quick reference guide for medical and surgical oncologists.

I have made every effort to ensure that the information contained in this book is accurate at the time of going to press.

Kefah Mokbel
*May 2005*

# About the author

**Professor Kefah Mokbel** is Consultant Breast and Endocrine Surgeon to St George's Hospital and a Professor at the Brunel Institute of Cancer Genetics and Pharmacogenomics. His main clinical interests include breast cancer surgery, including breast reconstruction and sentinel node biopsy, cosmetic breast surgery, including breast enlargement, breast reduction and mastopexy (breast lift). His main academic interests lie in the field of postgraduate education and research into molecular biology and the clinical management of breast cancer. He has had over 120 papers published in the medical literature and has written 10 books for postgraduate education. He is a member of the editorial board of several international medical journals. He also has an active research and teaching programme at St George's Hospital and Medical School, Brunel University (Institute of Cancer Genetics and Pharmacogenomics) and Kingston University (Life Sciences). He also supervises undergraduates and postgraduate research degrees. Professor Mokbel lectures nationally and internationally and teaches techniques of modern breast surgery, including skin-sparing mastectomy and immediate breast reconstruction, mammary ductoscopy and sentinel node biopsy.

# List of abbreviations

| | |
|---|---|
| ACTH | adrenocorticotrophic hormone |
| ADH | antidiuretic hormone |
| AFP | α-fetoprotein |
| AIDS | acquired immunodeficiency syndrome |
| ALL | acute lymphoblastic leukaemia |
| AML | acute myeloid leukaemia |
| BCC | basal-cell carcinoma |
| BCS | breast-conserving surgery |
| BMT | bone-marrow transplantation |
| BPH | benign prostatic hyperplasia |
| CBD | common bile duct |
| CEA | carcino-embryonic antigen |
| CIN | cervical intra-epithelial neoplasia |
| CIS | carcinoma *in situ* |
| CLL | chronic lymphocytic leukaemia |
| CML | chronic myelocytic leukaemia |
| CNS | central nervous system |
| CSF | cerebrospinal fluid |
| CT | computed tomography |
| CXR | chest X-ray |
| DCIS | ductal carcinoma *in situ* |
| DVT | deep vein thrombosis |
| EBV | Epstein–Barr virus |
| ECM | extracellular matrix |
| EEG | electroencephalogram |
| EGFR | epidermal growth factor receptor |
| ER | oestrogen receptor |
| ERCP | endoscopic retrograde cholangiopancreatography |
| ESR | erythrocyte sedimentation rate |
| EUA | examination under anaesthetic |

| | |
|---|---|
| FBC | full blood count/familial breast cancer |
| FIGO | International Federation of Gynaecology and Obstetrics |
| FISH | fluorescent *in situ* hybridisation |
| FNAC | fine-needle aspiration cytology |
| 5-FU | 5-fluorouracil |
| GI | gastrointestinal |
| Gy | gray |
| HBV | hepatitis B virus |
| HCC | hepatocellular carcinoma |
| HIV | human immunodeficiency virus |
| HPV | human papilloma virus |
| HSV | herpes simplex virus |
| IHC | immunohistochemistry |
| IM | intramuscularly |
| IV | intravenously |
| IVP | intravenous pyelography |
| IVU | intravenous urogram |
| KS | Kaposi's sarcoma |
| LABC | locally advanced breast cancer |
| LFT | liver function test |
| MBC | metastatic breast cancer |
| MEN | multiple endocrine neoplasia |
| MRI | magnetic resonance imaging |
| MTC | medullary thyroid carcinoma |
| MTH | medullary thyroid hyperplasia |
| NSCLC | non-small-cell lung cancer |
| OCP | oral contraceptive pill |
| PET | positron emission tomography |
| PSA | prostate-specific antigen |
| PTC | percutaneous transhepatic cholangiogram |
| PTH | parathyroid hormone |
| PUVA | psoralen with ultraviolet radiation A (long-wave) |
| RT | radiotherapy |
| SCC | squamous-cell carcinoma |
| SCLC | small-cell lung cancer |
| SNB | sentinel-node biopsy |
| TCC | transitional-cell carcinoma |
| TNM | tumour/node/metastasis staging |

| TSG | tumour suppressor gene |
| TSH | thyroid-stimulating hormone |
| TURP | transurethral resection of the prostate |
| U&Es | urea and electrolytes |
| USS | ultrasound scan |
| UV | ultraviolet |
| VMA | vanillyl mandelic acid |
| WBC | white blood count |
| 5-HT | 5-hydroxytryptophan |

# Principles of cancer screening

## Basic principles

- Screening may allow the detection of early disease in the asymptomatic population.
- The objective of screening, namely to reduce morbidity and mortality in those screened, must be balanced against the effectiveness of the programme.
- Screening may be applied to mass populations or to high-risk groups.

## Reliability of a screening test

- Sensitivity of the test is the proportion of individuals with the cancer who test positive. Sensitivity is a measure of false-negative results.
- Specificity of the test is the proportion of individuals without cancer who test negative. Specificity is a measure of false-positive results.
- Positive predictive value is the proportion of individuals with a positive test who have a diagnosis of cancer.
- Negative predictive value is the proportion of individuals with a negative test who do not have cancer.

# Biases within a screening programme

- Selection bias occurs when those attending for screening may have a better prognosis than, and are different from, the normal general population.
- Lead-time bias occurs when an earlier diagnosis is made by the screening test but the natural history is unaffected.
- Length bias occurs when patients with cancers are identified because they have slowly growing cancers leading to better survival.

# Attributes of a screening programme

- Ethically, the benefits of the programme should outweigh the risks associated with taking part in the programme.
- The cancer under study must have a long pre-clinical phase and the natural history should be well determined.
- Is there evidence from randomised controlled trials that treatment is effective?
- Does early treatment make a difference to outcome?
- Is the screening test reliable, acceptable to the population and economically viable?
- Is the morbidity associated with the screening test acceptable?

# Statistics

- The median value of a set of data is the central observation after the values have been ranked in order of size. That is, half of the data will have a value less than the median, and the other half of the data will have a value greater than the median. When the median is used as an indication of the central point of some data, then the centiles (e.g. quartiles, 95th centile, etc.) should be used as an indication of the shape or spread of the data.
- The mean is the sum of all the values in the population divided by the number of values in the population. When the mean is used as an indication of the central point of some data, then the standard deviation should be used as an indication of the shape or spread of the data.
- The null hypothesis ($H_0$) states that there is no difference between the data sets being compared and any apparent difference is due to chance.
- The $P$-value indicates the probability that the null hypothesis is correct. Therefore if it is a small value (e.g. < 0.05), the null hypothesis is rejected and the test is considered to be statistically significant (i.e. any difference that is observed is unlikely to be due to chance).
- A confidence interval gives an estimated range of values which is likely to include an unknown population parameter. The confidence level that is usually chosen for analysis is 95%. Confidence intervals are more informative than the simple results of hypothesis tests.
- In a normal distribution (which is symmetrical and bell-shaped), the mean and median are identical. A similar symmetrical, bell-shaped distribution is called the $t$ distribution with ($n$–1) degrees of freedom. The $t$ distribution also has a mean of 0, but the tails of the distribution are more spread out. The exact shape of the $t$ distribution depends on what are called degrees of freedom (df). The df are equal to the sample size minus 1.

**3**

Parametric tests such as the two-sample $t$-test and the paired $t$-test can be used with this type of data.

- Analysis of variance (ANOVA) is the term given to the method of analysing data from two or more groups.
- When the data are clearly not normally distributed, an alternative method is to use non-parametric techniques. These include the Mann–Whitney $U$-test and the Wilcoxon matched pairs test.
- The chi-squared test is a non-parametric test that is commonly used to assess frequency data and goodness of fit. It is preferable to use Fisher's exact test for $2 \times 2$ contingency table analysis instead of the chi-squared test.
- Correlation and regression methods examine the relationship between two continuous variables. Pearson's correlation coefficient ($r$) is a measure of the strength of the linear relationship between two parametric variables. A major assumption is the normal distribution of variables. If this is not met, the non-parametric equivalent, Spearman's rank correlation, should be used. The correlation coefficient $r$ can take any value between $-1$ and $+1$.
- The Cox regression method is used for modelling survival times. It is also called the proportional hazards model because it estimates the ratio of the risks (hazard ratio). As in any regression model, there are multiple predictor variables, such as prognostic parameters, whose individual contribution to the outcome is being assessed in the presence of the other predictor variables and the outcome variable. The model assumes that the underlying hazard rate is a function of the independent variables and that it is consistent over time.
- The survival curves are calculated using a procedure called the Kaplan–Meier method. Mathematically removing a patient from the curve at the end of their follow-up time is called 'censoring' the patient. Survival curves often have a tick mark at each point where a patient was censored. To determine the significance of the difference between survival times, the log rank test is used.
- The odds ratio (OR) is the ratio of the odds of the risk factor in a study group to those in a control group. The OR is used in retrospective case–control studies, whereas the relative risk

(RR) is the ratio of proportions in two groups which can be estimated in a prospective cohort study. These two ratios and the relative hazard ratio (or hazard ratio) are measures of the strength/magnitude of an association.

- A meta-analysis integrates the quantitative findings from separate but similar studies and provides a numerical estimate of the overall effect of interest.
- Absolute risk refers to the probability of an event occurring over a period of time. It is expressed as a cumulative incidence. It indicates the actual likelihood of an event occurring and provides a more realistic and comprehensible risk than the relative risk or odds ratio.
- A type I error is the kind of error that occurs if we reject the null hypothesis when it is true. If the null hypothesis is accepted when it is in fact wrong, this is a type II error. The statistical power of a test is equal to 1 minus the type II error. It is desirable for the power to exceed 80%.
- Survival statistics for cancer are usually expressed as 5-year survival or 10-year survival. Disease-free survival figures refer to everyone with that type of cancer who is alive and well without cancer recurrence.

# Drug pharmacology and clinical trials

## Basic principles

- Only 5–10% of all cancers are curable with currently available therapies – hence the need for drug development.
- Pharmacokinetics refers to drug absorption, distribution, metabolism and elimination. An understanding of pharmacokinetics may allow optimisation of effective drug delivery and hence of therapy.
- Pharmacodynamics is the study of the end-organ effects of the drug, and includes both the toxicity of the drug and its therapeutic actions.
- The dose, dose rate and schedule of drug administration all have a major influence on drug efficacy in oncology.
- A measure of drug exposure that is often used is the area under the plasma concentration versus time curve (the AUC).
- Relationships between pharmacokinetic (e.g. AUC) and pharmacodynamic (e.g. percentage change in platelet count) parameters have been described (e.g. for carboplatin), and can be used prospectively to minimise toxicity and potentially maximise activity.

## Clinical trials

- The development of new drugs has been based on pre-clinical *in-vitro* and *in-vivo* studies. This process has been accelerated by the use of X-ray crystallography and the design of active compounds based on the crystal structure of the target. Toxicology data from pre-clinical *in-vivo* studies are used to derive the starting dose for Phase I studies.

- Phase I clinical trials focus on drug toxicity and dosing schedules. Clinical pharmacokinetics are studied in detail, and pharmacokinetic analysis may be non-compartmental or compartmental, based on mathematical modelling. The primary aim of these studies is to determine the maximum tolerated dose (MTD) and the dose recommended for Phase II studies. This is achieved by means of dose escalations, which are determined through observed toxicities and pharmacokinetic analysis and pharmacodynamic studies relating drug toxicity to drug exposure (AUC). Phase I studies usually involve patients who have failed on previous treatment regimes, and usually small numbers of patients are treated at each dose level, the total number of patients involved in the trial tending to be around 30 on average. Patients are selected on the basis of strict eligibility criteria.
- Phase II trials use doses and schedules based on Phase I data. The aim of these trials is usually to determine efficacy based on tumour response. The studies select patients with specific tumour types and each trial assesses response. The study design may be based on fixed study subjects or on evaluations after subjects have been entered.
- Phase III trials are full-scale evaluations of the drug, involving randomisation, control groups, different study populations and treatment protocols.
- Phase IV involves post-marketing surveillance.

# 1 Oncogenesis

## Basic principles

- Carcinogenesis is a multi-step process.
- Initiation $\rightarrow$ promotion $\rightarrow$ cancer.
- Initiation is irreversible, whereas promotion is reversible.
- The effects of initiation are inheritable.
- DNA structural changes lead to tumour development.

## Host factors in carcinogenesis

- Immune system.
- Endogenous hormones.
- Genetic factors such as oncogenes and tumour suppressor genes.

## Environmental factors in carcinogenesis

- Radiation can cause DNA damage. It includes:
  - ionising radiation (e.g. X- and $\gamma$-rays, and $\alpha$- and $\beta$-particles)
  - non-ionising radiation (e.g. UV light).
- Chemical carcinogens. These include:
  - polycyclic hydrocarbons
  - aromatic amines
  - alkylating agents
  - blue asbestos
  - aflatoxins (hepatocellular carcinoma)
  - nicotine.
- Viruses. These include:
  - Epstein–Barr virus (EBV). This is a DNA oncogenic virus. It is a member of the herpes virus family. It is associated with Burkitt's lymphoma and nasopharyngeal carcinoma

- hepatitis B virus (HBV). The incidence of hepatocellular carcinoma is increased by 200-fold in chronic carriers of HBV
- human papilloma virus (HPV). This virus is associated with cervical cancer and epidermodysplasia verruciformis (multiple squamous-cell carcinomas of the skin)
- human T-cell leukaemia virus (HTLV-1). This is an RNA virus. It is associated with several malignancies, including leukaemias and lymphomas.

# Mechanisms of cancer pathogenesis

These include the following.

- Oncogenes are cancer-promoting genes which are derived from normal genes known as proto-oncogenes.
- Tumour suppressor genes restrict or repress cellular proliferation in normal cells. Their inactivation through somatic mutation or germ-line incorporation is associated with renal, colonic, breast, bladder and other cancers.
- DNA repair genes.
- Loss of imprinting.

# Oncogenes

- These are genes associated with neoplastic proliferation. The antecedent genes (known as *proto-oncogenes*) play an important physiological role in cellular growth.
- They can be classified into growth factors, growth factor receptors (e.g. erbB and fms), protein kinases (e.g. abl, src, mos and raf), signal transduction G proteins (e.g. H-, K- and N-ras) and nuclear proteins (e.g. c-myc, n-myc, fos, myb and jun).
- They are implicated in 20% of human tumours.
- Methods of activation include chromosomal rearrangement, gene amplification, point mutations and viral insertion.

# Tumour suppressor genes (TSGs)

- Loss or inactivation of TSGs can lead to neoplastic changes.
- p53 is a tumour suppressor gene located on chromosome 17p13.1. The normal form is known as the wild type. Loss of heterozygosity can lead to malignancy.
- Other examples of TSG include RB1, BRCA-1, BRCA-2 and DCC.

# DNA repair genes

- There are two major pathways of DNA repair, namely mismatch repair and nucleotide excision repair.
- Examples include xeroderma pigmentosa and the ataxia telangiectasia gene. Mutation of the latter (ATM) predisposes to leukaemia, lymphoma, and breast and skin cancers.

# Loss of imprinting

- Imprinting refers to the fact that the parental origin of the gene can affect its expression.

# 2 Tumour growth and metastases

Tumour cells can successfully metastasise if they have the ability to:

- regulate the production of proteases (by the tumour cells or surrounding stroma cells)
- regulate the production of adhesion molecules
- regulate the expression of major histocompatibility complex (MHC) units and escape immune surveillance, including natural killer cells
- regulate the process of clotting
- respond to cytokines and growth factors.

## The metalloproteinases

- There are at least eight members of this group of lytic enzymes that are responsible for the degradation of the extracellular matrix (ECM).
- They are secreted by the stromal elements or the tumour cells.

## Cadherins

- These are transmembrane glycoproteins which mediate haemophilic adhesions between cells.
- Down-regulation of E-cadherins is associated with dedifferentiation and metastasis of cells.

# Integrins

- These are transmembrane proteins which mediate cell adhesion to the ECM proteins and transmit signals.

# The sequential steps of metastasis

These include the following.

- Malignant transformation.
- Cell proliferation resulting in a primary tumour mass.
- Angiogenesis when primary tumour exceeds 2 mm in diameter.
- Detachment of cells from primary tumour in association with down-regulation of E-cadherins.
- Detached tumour cells interact with ECM by integrins.
- Motility of tumour cells is stimulated by scatter factor secreted by fibroblasts or by motility factors secreted by the tumour cells.
- Metalloproteinases secreted by tumour cells or stromal fibroblasts degrade ECM and allow invasion of blood vessels and lymphatics.
- Within blood vessels/lymphatics some tumour cells are attacked by T-cells, while others escape immune surveillance due to lack of or altered MHC units.
- Tumour cells adhere to endothelial cells via integrins, intracellular adhesion molecules, selectins, CD44 and other adhesion molecules.
- Tumour cell invasion of target tissues is facilitated by metalloproteinases which degrade ECM.

# TNM classification

- Solid tumours can be staged according to the TNM system.
- The TNM staging system is a systematic method of describing the size, location and spread of a tumour.
- T describes the primary tumour according to its size and location (T0, T1, T2, etc.).

- N indicates whether the cancer has spread to the regional lymph nodes (i.e. N0 or N1).
- M indicates whether the cancer has spread to distant organs in the body (M0 or M1).
- X indicates that the status is not known (e.g. MX means that we do not know whether metastatic disease to other organs is present).
- Group staging is frequently used to include several TNM stages in one group (e.g. stage I can include T1N0M0, T2N0M0 and T1N1M0 tumours).

# Gene expression profiling

Gene expression profiling is a new microarray-based technology that determines the expression of a large number of genes in tissue specimens simultaneously. This analytical method is currently being investigated as an emerging diagnostic and prognostic tool for several human cancers. An important assumption behind this research is that the constellation of multiple genes will be a more accurate predictor of clinical outcome than any single gene alone. These new technologies are more potent when coupled with advanced bioinformatics analysis.

# Proteomics

Proteomics is the analysis of proteins present in the organism in normal and pathological conditions using microarray-based technology, mass spectrometry and advanced bioinformatics analysis. This allows scientists to identify the proteomic biosignatures of human cancer in both serum and tissue specimens. The potential clinical applications include diagnosis, tailoring of therapy, prediction of outcome and the identification of new targets for therapy.

# 3 Principles of chemotherapy

## The cell cycle

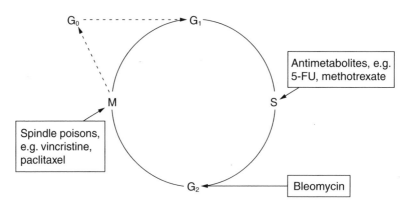

**Figure 1**   The cell cycle. M = mitosis phase, $G_1$ = gap 1, S = synthesis phase, $G_2$ = gap 2, $G_0$ = resting phase.

- The duration of the cell cycle is approximately 48 hours.
- Stimulatory signals come from cyclins (cyclins D and E in the $G_1$ phase, cyclin A in the S phase and cyclin B in the $G_2$ and M phases). Inhibitory signals come from tumour suppressor genes (e.g. p53 and RB1).
- Cytotoxic drugs kill tumour cells and normal cells, but tumour cells have a greater sensitivity to these drugs or a reduced ability to repair cytotoxic damage.
- Chemotherapy agents can be cycle specific (e.g. alkylating and intercalating) or phase specific (e.g. spindle poisons and antimetabolites).

# Classification of cytotoxic drugs

- Alkylating agents:
  - chemically react with the structure forming methyl cross-bridges between the two strands of DNA base pairs. This prevents the DNA strands from coming apart during mitosis, and division therefore fails
  - examples include nitrogen mustards, melphalan, chlorambucil, cyclophosphamide, busulfan, nitrosoureas, platinum and dacarbazine.
- Antimetabolites:
  - inhibit the formation of essential nucleic acids, thus interfering with DNA/RNA synthesis and causing cell death
  - examples include methotrexate, 5-fluorouracil (5-FU), cytosine, arabinoside and purine analogues
  - folinic acid can be given to rescue cells from the effect of methotrexate.
- Anti-tumour antibiotics:
  - anthracyclines include doxorubicin, daunorubicin and epirubicin. These drugs intercalate between base pairs of DNA, causing DNA damage. Mitoxantrone is structurally related to this group of drugs
  - bleomycin – this drug is $G_2$ specific
  - mitomycin C – this acts as an alkylating agent and generates free radicals capable of causing DNA damage
  - actinomycin D – this intercalates between guanine and cytosine, thus inhibiting DNA/RNA synthesis
  - platinum analogues (cisplatin and carboplatin).
- Plant-derived cytotoxic drugs:
  - vinca alkaloids. Vincristine, vinblastine and vindesine inhibit the formation of mitotic spindles by binding to tubulin
  - epidophyllotoxins (e.g. etoposide). These drugs interfere with topoisomerase II enzymes, causing DNA damage during the S phase
  - paclitaxel (Taxol) inhibits mitosis by promoting a disorganised and stabilised assembly of microtubules. It is a new drug and is mainly used in the treatment of breast and ovarian cancers. Docetaxel (Taxotere) is a similar drug.

- Other drugs:
  - dacarbazine is an alkylating agent used in the treatment of melanoma
  - procarbazine is used to treat Hodgkin's lymphoma.

# Chemotherapy protocols

- Combinations are usually used.
- Pulsed or intermittent therapy is frequently used in order to allow a larger dose to be given.
- High-dose chemotherapy can be given with the use of haematopoietic growth factors, stem cell support or autologous bone marrow transplantation in order to counteract myelosuppression.

# Mechanisms of drug resistance

- Increased concentrations of target enzymes (e.g. doxorubicin, epirubicin, paclitaxel, vincristine).
- Reduced uptake by tumour cells (e.g. daunorubicin).
- Increased activity of salvage pathways (e.g. antimetabolites).
- Detoxification.
- Improved DNA repair mechanisms by target cells.
- Impairment of activation or increased inactivation of the drug.

# Biological therapy

- Recent advances in molecular biology have led to the development of numerous biological therapies.
- Herceptin is a recombinant humanised monoclonal antibody that binds and blocks the growth receptor HER2. It has been shown to be effective in patients with metastatic breast cancer overexpressing HER2. Phase II trials are currently in progress in patients with ovarian cancer.
- Rituximab is an anti-CD20 monoclonal antibody which seems to be effective in the treatment of refractory indolent lymphoma and hairy cell leukaemia.

- Angiogenesis inhibitors include angiotensin, endostatin and epidermal growth factor receptor (EGFR) antagonists. These agents are currently being evaluated.
- Immunotherapy.

# 4 Principles of radiotherapy

## Basic principles

- X-rays are the commonest type of ionising radiation used in clinical practice. They are produced artificially by accelerating electrons (linear accelerators) using microwave energy, resulting in the production of therapeutic megavolt beams.
- Gamma rays are similar to X-rays but arise from the decay of radioactive isotopes.
- Ionising radiation causes irreversible DNA damage either directly or indirectly by generating toxic free radicals. The DNA damage, which is oxygen dependent, is the most important factor in cell killing.
- Radiotherapy dose is expressed in grays or centigrays (1 Gy = 100 cGy), and describes the energy absorbed per unit mass of tissue.
- Fractionation allows a higher degree of radiation to be given.

## Clinical applications

- Cancer patients are treated either by external beam radiation (linear accelerator or cobalt machine) or by insertion of a radioactive material into body tissues (interstitial radiotherapy) or cavities (intracavity radiotherapy).
- Radiotherapy can be palliative or curative. It can be combined with other treatment modalities such as surgery and chemotherapy. Pre-operative radiotherapy may be given in order to render a tumour operable. Post-operative radiotherapy is used mainly to reduce the rate of local recurrence.

- The effects of radiotherapy depend on the dose, the tumour size, the tumour proliferation rate, hypoxia, tumour radio-sensitivity, the patient's performance, the presence of anaemia and vascular disease.

# Side-effects

- Early side-effects include mucositis, alopecia, skin erythema, nausea, vomiting, enteritis and bone marrow suppression. These side-effects are reversible and can be managed symptomatically.
- Late side-effects include spinal cord myelitis, pneumonitis, strictures, telangiectasia and secondary cancers. Approximately 3% of patients develop a second cancer 15 years after treatment.

# 5 Cancer of the lip

## Epidemiology

- The incidence is higher among Caucasians (compared with blacks), smokers and outdoor workers.
- Cancer of the lip accounts for 25% of oral malignancies.

## Pathology

- Smoking (especially pipe smoking) and solar radiation are important aetiological factors.
- Squamous-cell carcinoma (SCC) is the commonest histological type. Basal-cell carcinoma is occasionally seen.
- Around 92% of lesions occur on the lower lip, 5% occur on the upper lip and 3% at the angle of the mouth.
- Submandibular nodes are the usual sites for metastases.

## Investigation

- Limited surgical biopsy under local anaesthetic.
- Fine-needle aspiration cytology (FNAC) of enlarged lymph nodes.

## Treatment

- Surgery and radiotherapy are equally effective.
- Surgical defects following adequate excision can be reconstructed using local flaps (from the opposite lip) or closed primarily if small. Local reconstruction aims to maximise the functional and cosmetic outcomes.
- The cure rate is 90%.

# 6 Oral cancer

## Epidemiology

- It accounts for 4% of all cancers (India has the highest incidence).
- Peak incidence is in the age group 50–70 years.
- It is more common in men.
- The tongue is the commonest site.

## Pathology

- Squamous-cell carcinoma (SCC) accounts for 90% of all cases.
- Adenocarcinoma accounts for 3% of cases.
- Kaposi's sarcoma, lymphoma and melanoma are rare.
- The TNM system is used for staging.

## Aetiology

Risk factors include:

- smoking and chewing tobacco
- alcohol
- infections (syphilis, candidiasis and herpes virus)
- immunosuppression
- industrial hazards (textile workers, nickel exposure)
- oncogenes (ras, p53, L-myc and C-myc)
- leukoplakia
- erythroplakia.

## Clinical presentation

- Ulcerating lesions.

- Exophytic lesions.
- Induration.
- Swelling.
- Pain.
- Pathological mandibular fractures.
- Paraesthesia along the inferior alveolar nerve distribution.
- Lymphadenopathy in the head and neck region.

# Investigations

- Exfoliative cytology.
- Surgical biopsy including a margin of healthy tissue.
- CT and MRI.
- FNAC of enlarged lymph nodes.
- Plain radiograph of adjacent teeth may be useful.

# Treatment

- SCC of the anterior two-thirds of the tongue.
  - This can be treated with surgical excision (with a 1 mm margin) or radiotherapy.
  - Large surgical defects can be reconstructed using split-thickness skin grafts, local skin flaps (forehead or delto-pectoral), myocutaneous flaps (pectoralis major or trapezius) or free flaps (microvascular anastomosis).
- SCC in the floor of the mouth.
  - If the alveolar process is involved then wide local excision with reconstruction (local or free flaps) is appropriate.
  - If the alveolar process is not involved, then radiotherapy is the treatment of choice.
- SCC on the mandibular alveolus is treated with surgical excision and reconstruction using bone grafting or a free flap utilising the underlying bone (radial forearm flap).
- SCC of the buccal mucosa is treated with surgical resection and the defect is reconstructed with a local or free flap.

- SCC on the upper jaw is treated with surgical excision and reconstruction using a prosthetic appliance lined with skin graft if necessary.
- Supraomohyoid or modified radical neck dissection may be necessary, depending on lymph node involvement.
- Post-operative adjuvant radiotherapy or chemotherapy may be necessary.

# Prognosis

- The overall 5-year survival rate of patients with carcinoma of the tongue is approximately 40%. Posterior location and advanced stage are adverse prognostic parameters.

# 7 Cancer of the salivary glands

## Epidemiology

- The incidence is 1.5 per 100 000 per year.
- Around 70% of the lesions occur in the parotid gland (20% are malignant).

## Aetiology

- Malignant transformation of a pleomorphic adenoma.
- Radiation.
- Association with breast cancer.

## Pathology

- The grade (high grade or low grade) is more important than the histological type (acinic cell, mucoepidermoid or carcinoma) in predicting behaviour and prognosis.

## Clinical presentation

- Swelling (rate of growth depends upon grade of tumour).
- Facial nerve palsy (parotid tumours).
- Sensory loss in anterior two-thirds of the tongue (submandibular tumours).
- Trismus and pain along the trigeminal nerve distribution.
- Lymphadenopathy (25% of cases).

# Investigations

- Core biopsy or FNAC.
- Open biopsy.
- CT or MRI.
- Staging investigations include CXR, thoracic CT and bone scan.

# Management

- Surgical excision for low-grade tumours.
- Surgical excision followed by radiotherapy for high-grade tumours.
- The facial nerve may be sacrificed in some cases.
- Neck dissection is indicated in the presence of lymph node metastases (confirmed by FNAC).
- Pre-operative radiotherapy followed by surgery for locally advanced tumours.
- Radiotherapy alone has a local control rate of 30% in patients with locally advanced tumours.
- Plastic reconstruction may be performed using pectoralis major, trapezius and latissimus dorsi myocutaneous flaps or a radial forearm free flap.

# Prognosis

- For low-grade tumours the 10-year survival rate is 90%.
- For high-grade tumours the 10-year survival rate is 25%.
- In addition to grade, histopathological subtype, tumour stage and margin status significantly influence the prognosis.

# 8 Retinoblastoma

## Epidemiology

- The incidence is 1 per 15 000 live births.
- It accounts for 3% of all childhood malignancies.
- The incidence is increasing. It has doubled in the last 40 years.

## Aetiology

- Most cases are sporadic.
- Some cases are inherited in an autosomal dominant fashion. Sporadic bilateral retinoblastoma and familial retinoblastoma are inheritable.
- The retinoblastoma (Rb) gene is a growth suppressor gene. Its product has a general suppressive function in the cell cycle.

## Pathology

- The tumour usually consists of undifferentiated and small cells with deeply staining nuclei and scanty cytoplasm.
- The tumour is usually multifocal.
- The commonest mode of metastasis is via the bloodstream to bone marrow, liver, lungs and lymph nodes.
- The tumour is classified according to the Reese–Ellsworth system into five groups (I–V).

## Clinical features

- The tumour usually presents before the age of 2 years.
- 'White pupil' is the commonest presentation.

- Other features include strabismus, glaucoma, defect in visual fixation and inflammatory changes within the eye.
- Ophthalmological assessment is required in such cases. Surgical biopsy is not recommended.

# Investigations

- Full blood count (FBC), bone scan and CXR.
- Orbital CT or MRI.
- Analysis of CSF if intracranial spread is suspected.

# Management

- Cryosurgery or photocoagulation for very small lesions.
- Brachytherapy (for lesions measuring 3–10 mm) using radioactive cobalt.
- External beam radiation (35–40 Gy over 4 weeks) for large lesions and for lesions near the optic disc and macula.
- Eye enucleation for tumours that are unresponsive to conservative management and for tumour that is occupying most of the eye and infiltrating the optic nerve. Post-operative radiotherapy may be given in such cases.
- Chemotherapy may be used for extra-ocular disease and to reduce the bulk of primary disease in order to allow conservative treatment (chemoreductive neoadjuvant therapy). Effective agents include vincristine, actinomycin D, doxorubicin, methotrexate and cyclophosphamide.
- An orbital integrated implant can be placed after enucleation, and provides acceptable prosthesis motility and appearance.
- Genetic counselling is an important part of management.

# Prognosis

- The cure rate for stages I and II is 100%.
- The cure rate for stages IV and V is 75%.
- The overall mortality is 10%.

# 9 Laryngeal cancer

## Epidemiology

- Laryngeal cancer accounts for 2–3% of all malignant disease.
- The male:female ratio is 10:1.
- The disease occurs exclusively in smokers.
- The peak age of onset is 60 years.

## Pathology

- Squamous-cell carcinoma accounts for most cases.
- Adenoid cystic carcinoma and sarcoma are rare.
- Laryngeal cancer can be classified into four types according to site of origin:
  - glottic (60%)
  - supraglottic (30%)
  - subglottic (5%)
  - marginal (5%).
- The disease spread is local initially.
- Lymphatic spread is to deep cervical lymph nodes.
- Pulmonary metastases are occasionally seen.

## Clinical features

- Hoarseness is the main symptom of the disease.
- Other symptoms include:
  - dysphagia
  - earache
  - dyspnoea
  - haemoptysis.

# Investigations

- Microlaryngoscopy and biopsy.
- CXR.
- CT to define the extent of the disease.

# Treatment

- Glottic tumours.
  - Carcinoma *in situ* can be treated by local excision of the involved mucosa. This can be performed endoscopically.
  - T1 and T2 lesions can be effectively treated with radiotherapy. The resulting voice quality is better than after partial (vertical) laryngectomy. Salvage surgery in the form of partial or total laryngectomy is performed in cases where failure occurs with radiotherapy treatment.
  - Tumours involving the contralateral cord can be treated by total laryngectomy. Post-operative radiotherapy may be given.
- Early supraglottic tumours are treated by pre-operative radiotherapy and subsequent total laryngectomy.
- Advanced supraglottic, subglottic and glottic tumours are treated by means of radiotherapy, chemotherapy and/or surgery.
- Lymph node dissection is indicated if there is evidence of nodal spread (e.g. positive cytology).
- Following total laryngectomy, 60% of patients develop reasonable oesophageal speech. Many patients are now provided with a valve fitted to a tracheopharyngeal fistula. Phonation is produced by occluding the tracheostomy with a finger.
- Tracheostomy care training, speech therapy and social support are important aspects of management.
- Recent evidence indicates that induction chemotherapy can achieve an excellent response and increased rates of larynx preservation in patients with locally advanced disease.

# Prognosis

- The cure rates for T1 and T2 lesions are 90% and 65%, respectively.
- The 5-year survival rate for T3 tumours is 25%.

# 10 Lung cancer

## Epidemiology

- This is the commonest form of cancer in Western countries.
- The male:female ratio is 4:1.

## Aetiology

- Prolonged exposure to cigarette smoke is the most important aetiological factor. This increases the risk by 53-fold.
- Asbestos exposure.
- Industrial pollution (e.g. coal and tar fumes, diesel exhausts, nickel, zinc, beryllium, radon).
- Occupational exposure to nickel, chromium, iron oxide or arsenicals.
- Pre-existing lung disease such as old TB and fibrosis (scar carcinomas).

## Pathology

- Squamous-cell carcinoma (which accounts for 40% of cases) tends to arise proximally in large bronchi. It is associated with loss of heterozygosity of the p53 gene.
- In small-cell lung cancer (20% of cases) neurosecretory granules are often present and produce various hormones (e.g. calcitonin, ADH, ACTH, PTH). It is associated with over-expression of C-myc and loss of heterozygosity of the p53 gene.
- Adenocarcinoma (15–50% of cases) tends to arise in scars and peripheral sites. It is more common in women. It may be bronchoalveolar or bronchoacinar. It is less strongly associated with smoking than the other types.

- Large-cell carcinoma (10% of cases).
- Mixed histologies (15% of cases).
- Carcinoid tumours (< 1% of cases).
- Sarcoma (< 1% of cases).

Carcinoma of the bronchus spreads by local invasion and by lymphatic and haematogenous routes.

# Clinical features

- The commonest symptoms are haemoptysis, cough, dyspnoea and chest pain.
- Other features include:
  - hoarseness
  - pleural effusion
  - phrenic nerve palsy
  - pneumonia
  - pulmonary collapse
  - dysphagia
  - stridor
  - superior vena cava obstruction (SVCO)
  - Pancoast's tumour
  - mass in the neck
  - bone metastases
  - anorexia
  - weight loss
  - hypercalcaemia
  - SIADH (syndrome of inappropriate ADH secretion)
  - Cushing's syndrome
  - features of metastases to brain and intraperitoneal cavity.

# Investigations

- CXR.
- Exfoliative sputum cytology (four specimens).
- Bronchoscopy and biopsy.

- CT scanning to guide thoracic needle biopsy and to define tumour extent.
- MRI to assess spread to cardiovascular organs.
- Mediastinoscopy to assess extent of disease.
- Other investigations include:
  - FBC
  - serum biochemistry
  - bone scan
  - liver USS
  - brain CT
  - lymph node biopsy
  - pleural fluid cytology, etc.

# Staging (TNM system)

- Stage I:
  - T1,2N0M0
  - T1N1M0.
- Stage II:
  - T2N1M0.
- Stage III:
  - any T3
  - any N2
  - any M1.

# Treatment and prognosis

- Non-small-cell lung cancer (NSCLC).
  - Less than 50% of cases are resectable at the time of diagnosis.
  - Operable cases may be treated by wedge excision (for localised peripheral tumours), lobectomy (for more centrally located tumours) or pneumectomy (for tumours of the main bronchus where more than one lobe is involved or the hilum is involved).

- The 5-year survival rate for resectable tumours is 55% for stage I, 30% for stage II and 18% for stage III. T1 squamous-cell tumours have the best survival rate (80%).
- Radical radiotherapy (60 Gy over 6 weeks) is indicated in patients who have resectable tumours but who are unfit for or refuse surgery. The 5-year survival rate is 10%.
- Palliative radiotherapy to relieve troublesome symptoms in patients with inoperable disease.
- Chemotherapy has a limited role in localised NSCLC. The benefit is estimated to be 5%. Drugs used include taxanes, mitomycin, cisplatin, cyclophosphamide, doxorubicin, etc. The drugs may be given in combination before or after radiotherapy or surgery.
- Small-cell lung cancer (SCLC).
  - The majority of patients present with extensive disease.
  - Radiotherapy is the mainstay of treatment for loco-regional disease and metastases. The primary tumour response rate is 80% with 50 Gy over 5 weeks.
  - Combination chemotherapy (doxorubicin, etoposide and cyclophosphamide) is indicated in fit patients.
  - The 2-year survival rate for limited disease is 15%.

# Biological therapy

- Recent clinical trials have failed to demonstrate any superiority for Iressa (an EGFR antagonist) compared with placebo in patients with locally advanced or metastatic NSCLC that is refractory to chemotherapy.
- Introduction of the wild-type p53 plus a viral vector (e.g. an adenovirus) into advanced pulmonary tumours is currently being investigated. The initial results are encouraging.

# 11 Breast cancer

## Epidemiology

- Breast cancer is the leading cause of death among women.
- The lifetime risk is approximately 10%.
- The average incidence is 65 per 100 000 individuals per year.

## Aetiology

- Risk factors include:
  - early menarche (the relative risk is 1.5)
  - late menopause (early menopause is protective)
  - obesity after the menopause (pre-menopausal obesity is protective)
  - nulliparity (increases risk by 30%)
  - late pregnancy (e.g. after the age of 35 years)
  - benign breast disease, especially atypical epithelial hyperplasia
  - oral contraceptives
  - hormone replacement therapy (seems to increase the risk by 35% after use for 5 years)
  - family history of breast cancer. The risk is particularly high in the first-degree relatives of patients with early onset of breast cancer (age < 45 years) and/or bilateral breast cancer
  - alcohol consumption is associated with increased risk
  - ionising radiation. The risk increases with radiation dose. Exposure during the second decade has a maximal risk. The latency period is 15–20 years
  - elevated serum insulin-like growth factor type 1 (IGF-1).

# Screening

- Screening mammography is recommended for:
  - all women aged 50–69 years (every 2 years)
  - all women aged 40–49 years (every 12–18 months)
  - all women with a previous history of breast cancer or a significant family history of breast cancer (annual mammography).
- Screening mammography has been shown to reduce breast cancer mortality by 30% in women aged over 50 years.
- There is increasing evidence that MRI is effective in screening high-risk young women with dense breasts.

# Pathology

- Ductal carcinoma *in situ* (DCIS) is confined to the duct-lobular units without breaching the basement membrane. It is subclassified into:
  - low nuclear grade, with or without necrosis
  - intermediate nuclear grade, with or without necrosis
  - high nuclear grade, with or without necrosis.

The risk of developing into invasive cancer is greatest for high-grade DCIS associated with necrosis.

- Lobular carcinoma *in situ* (LCIS). This is a marker of increased risk of developing breast cancer. The risk of developing invasive cancer is approximately 25% after 20 years. The invasive lesion may be ductal.
- Infiltrating ductal carcinoma. This is the commonest type.
- Infiltrating lobular carcinoma. This type is associated with a higher incidence of bilateral breast cancer, and its extent is frequently underestimated by breast imaging.
- Colloid carcinoma:
  - accounts for 5% of breast cancers
  - has a good prognosis.
- Tubular carcinoma has an excellent prognosis.
- Cribriform carcinoma is rare and has a good prognosis.

- Papillary carcinoma is rare and has a good prognosis.
- Medullary carcinoma has a good prognosis and is associated with a family history of breast cancer.
- Paget's disease of the breast, in which there is skin infiltration by large pale-staining malignant cells.
- Inflammatory carcinoma accounts for 2% of all cases. There is erythema, tenderness and invasion of the dermal lymphatics by tumour cells. It has a poor prognosis.
- Squamous-cell carcinoma:
  - is a rare tumour and usually lacks hormone receptors
  - the prognosis is similar to that of infiltrating ductal cell carcinoma
  - a primary extra-mammary lesion should be excluded.

# Clinical features

- Symptoms include:
  - breast lump (85% of cases)
  - pain (5%)
  - nipple retraction (5%)
  - nipple discharge (2%)
  - Paget's disease (5%)
  - axillary mass (1%)
  - skin changes (1%)
  - distant metastases.
- Clinical examination usually reveals a solid mass which may be ill-defined and fixed to overlying/underlying structures.
- The loco-regional lymph nodes, thoracic spine and abdomen should be examined in the search for metastases.
- Breast cancer may present as an impalpable mammographic abnormality during screening. DCIS accounts for 20% of screen-detected cancers and usually presents as pleomorphic microcalcifications.

# Investigations

- FNAC:
  - has a high specificity (> 98%) in the hands of experienced cytologists
  - cannot distinguish between infiltrating and *in-situ* lesions
  - can be performed stereotactically and can be ultrasound guided.
- Core biopsy:
  - specificity approaches 100%
  - is indicated if neoadjuvant chemotherapy is considered, if mastectomy is planned, for impalpable microcalcification (under stereotactic guidance) and if FNAC is equivocal.
- Mammography:
  - signs of malignancy, including spiculated masses, circumscribed masses, microcalcifications, stellate lesions, parenchymal distortions, skin tethering and retraction and nipple inversion.
- Ultrasound examination (with or without Doppler).
- Cytological analysis of scrape smear (of nipple) and nipple discharge.
- MRI of the breast is useful for estimating the extent of disease and assessing response to neoadjuvant therapy.
- Investigations for suspected metastatic disease include:
  - FBC, serum biochemistry and CXR (all patients)
  - liver USS and bone scan for patients with symptoms/signs suggestive of metastatic disease, abnormal serum biochemistry or grossly involved axillary nodes
  - bone MRI if bone scan is equivocal
  - computed tomography (CT) and/or positron emission tomography (PET) for suspected lung metastases.

# Management

- Localised invasive breast cancer.
  - Breast-conserving surgery (BCS) entails wide local excision of the tumour and axillary dissection. The sentinel-node

biopsy (SNB) using the dual localisation technique should be considered in all patients with clinically node-negative early breast cancer, and if the SNB is positive for malignancy on intra-operative frozen section, complete axillary clearance is performed.

– Mastectomy is indicated for central tumours, multi-centric disease, Paget's disease of the breast, large tumours (> 4 cm in diameter), or if the patient requests mastectomy. Immediate breast reconstruction should be offered to fit patients who are undergoing mastectomy.

– Adjuvant radiotherapy (RT) is indicated after BCS (all cases). Post-mastectomy RT is indicated if the tumour is node-positive (four or more positive nodes) or incompletely excised.

– Adjuvant tamoxifen is indicated if the tumour is ER and/or progesterone receptor (PgR) positive.

– Adjuvant cytotoxic chemotherapy (anthracycline based) is indicated for fit patients with node-positive disease or with high-risk (e.g. ER-negative, grade III and/or large size) node-negative disease.

- DCIS.
  – Wide local excision with adequate margins is the mainstay of management.

  – Adjuvant RT is indicated after BCS, especially if the tumour is large in size, of high grade or close to the excision margins.

  – Mastectomy is indicated for multi-centric disease, large lesions, Paget's disease or if the patient requests mastectomy. No adjuvant RT is required after mastectomy. Immediate breast reconstruction should be offered.

  – Tamoxifen is not currently indicated for DCIS. It may be considered if DCIS is of high grade, large size and close to or involving the excision margins, especially in women younger than 50 years (when no further surgery is possible).

  – Formal axillary-node dissection is not indicated for DCIS. The sentinel-node biopsy may be considered for high-risk DCIS treated by mastectomy.

- Locally advanced breast cancer (LABC).
  – Initial treatment consists of systemic therapy (endocrine or cytotoxic) and/or RT. Subsequent treatment includes BCS or total mastectomy.

- Post-menopausal women with ER- and/or PgR-positive LABC can be treated with an aromatase inhibitor (e.g. letrozole or anastrozole).
- Pre-menopausal women with ER- and/or PgR-positive LABC can be treated with goserelin.
- ER- and PgR-negative LABC is treated by cytotoxic therapy (e.g. taxanes and anthracyclines).
- USS, MRI and/or Ki-67 expression can be used to monitor response.

- Metastatic breast cancer (MBC).
  - ER and/or PgR positive MBC is treated with an aromatase inhibitor (anastrozole, letrozole or exemestane) in post-menopausal patients, and with goserelin (plus tamoxifen or an aromatase inhibitor) in pre-menopausal patients.
  - Cytotoxic therapy (taxanes and anthracyclines) is indicated for ER- and PgR-negative disease. Xeloda is an oral therapy that seems to improve survival when added to Taxotere.
  - Herceptin, either as monotherapy or in combination with Taxol, is indicated for HER2-positive (immunohistochemistry (IHC) score of 3 or more or FISH positive) disease.
  - Bisphosphonates are indicated for multiple bone metastases.
  - RT is indicated for painful localised bone or brain metastases.
  - Palliative measures include analgesia, thoracostomy tubes and pleurodesis, and drainage of ascites.

- Breast care counsellors play an important part in the management of patients, and provide psychological support and information.

- All patients who are undergoing mastectomy should be offered immediate breast reconstruction (IBR). If IBR is considered, then skin-sparing mastectomy combined with a mammary implant and/or a myocutaneous flap achieves an excellent cosmetic result without compromising oncological safety. The flap can be either a latissimus dorsi (LD) or a transverse rectus abdominus myocutaneous (TRAM) flap. TRAM flaps can be either conventional or free transfer, and do not usually require a prosthesis. Muscle-sparing free-transfer flaps based on the deep inferior epigastric perforator (DIEP) are increasing in popularity. The latter technique should be delayed if possible in cases where post-mastectomy RT is indicated.

# Prognosis

- Axillary-node status is the best single predictor of prognosis.
- Other prognostic parameters include tumour size, tumour grade, ER status, lymphovascular invasion, expression of p53, Ki-67 and HER2, microvessel density and bone-marrow micrometastases.
- The 5-year disease-free survival rate is 95% for stage 0 (DCIS), 85% for stage I, 70% for stage II, 50% for stage III and 15% for stage IV.
- Around 98% of DCIS lesions are cured by mastectomy.

# Follow-up

- Six-monthly review for 2 years and then annual review for 3 years.
- Annual mammography.

# Familial breast cancer (FBC)

- This accounts for 5% of all breast cancers.
- Genes responsible include the BRCA-1 gene (also responsible for ovarian cancer) on 17q21, the BRCA-2 gene on 13q12–13, the p53 gene on 17p13, the ataxia telangiectasia gene on 11q23 and the androgen-receptor gene on the X-chromosome.
- FBC can be treated with breast-conserving surgery plus RT.
- Prophylactic bilateral mastectomy can reduce the risk by 90% in patients carrying BRCA genes. Tamoxifen and ovarian ablation are also likely to reduce the risk.

# Recent advances and future prospects

- Third-generation aromatase inhibitors (letrozole, anastrozole and exemestane) are becoming the drugs of choice for the treatment of advanced post-menopausal breast cancer which is ER- and/or PgR-positive as first-line and second-line agents.
- The ATAC trial has recently reported its preliminary results after a median follow-up of 47 months. It has demonstrated that adjuvant anastrozole is superior to tamoxifen in reducing the risk of local recurrence and preventing contralateral breast cancer in post-menopausal women with hormone-sensitive disease. Although further follow-up is required, anastrozole can be used as an adjuvant therapy if tamoxifen is contra-indicated (e.g. if there is a history of deep vein thrombosis and endometrial hyperplasia/cancer) or cannot be tolerated. Bisphos-phonates, vitamin D and calcium can be added to anastrozole in women who are at risk of osteoporosis.
- Faslodex (250 mg IM once monthly) is a selective oestrogen-receptor down-regulator. Recent phase III clinical trials have demonstrated that it is at least as effective as anastrozole in post-menopausal patients with advanced disease who relapsed or progressed on prior endocrine therapy. In the first-line setting it is equivalent to tamoxifen, except in patients with tumours that are ER- and PgR-positive, where Faslodex seems to be superior.
- Letrozole (an aromatase inhibitor) has recently been shown to be an effective neoadjuvant agent in post-menopausal women with ER- and/or PgR-positive tumours. The drug was found to be superior in efficacy to tamoxifen, and increased the rate of BCS in a phase III study. It is significantly more effective than tamoxifen in patients with HER2 disease.
- Microarray gene profiling, which allows the identification of thousands of genes, is likely to enter clinical practice within the next five years. This new technology may improve the prog-nosis prediction and guide therapy.

- Digital mammography seems to achieve better-quality images than conventional mammography. This new technology also facilitates image storage and transmission, and allows the use of computer-aided detection.
- Fibre-optic ductoscopy seems to be an effective diagnostic tool in patients with pathological nipple discharge. It may have a role in guiding breast cancer surgery and cancer detection.
- There is increasing evidence that cyclo-oxygenase type 2 (COX-2) plays an important role in mammary carcinogenesis and angiogenesis. Selective COX-2 inhibitors may therefore prove to be effective in the treatment and prevention of breast cancer. Clinical trials are currently in progress.
- Aromatase inhibitors (e.g. letrozole) have a potential role in extended adjuvant therapy after 5 years of tamoxifen treatment and in sequential therapy after 2–3 years of tamoxifen treatment.
- Proteomics is likely to have a role in breast cancer detection.
- Electrical impedance and conductance and thermovascular measurements may have a role in cancer detection.
- Localised radiotherapy may prove as effective as and even replace whole breast irradiation.

# 12 Oesophageal cancer

## Epidemiology

- The incidence ranges from 3 to 180 per 100 000 per year, depending upon geographical location.
- There is a geographical clustering in certain parts of Asia and Africa.
- The male:female ratio is 7:1.
- The incidence of adenocarcinoma (mostly located distally) has been increasing.

## Aetiology

Risk factors include:

- Barrett's oesophagus (13% risk). High-grade dysplasia is associated with the highest risk
- achalasia
- corrosive strictures
- diverticular disease of the oesophagus
- Plummer–Vinson syndrome
- smoking, alcohol consumption, the rubber industry, vitamin C deficiency, human papilloma virus (a minor role), zinc deficiency and tylosis.

# Pathology

- In Asia, 80% of carcinomas are of the squamous-cell type and 15% are adenocarcinomas. The middle third is the commonest location.
- In Western countries, 45% of carcinomas are adenocarcinomas and 50% are squamous-cell carcinomas. Lesions of the lower oesophagus and cardia are more common in these countries.

# Clinical presentation

- Dysphagia (95% of cases).
- Regurgitation (45%).
- Weight loss (40%).
- Cough (25%).
- Pain (20%).
- Hoarse voice (20%).
- Dyspnoea (5%).
- Haemoptysis (5%).
- Haematemesis (5%).
- Neck mass (5%).
- Anaemia.

# Physical examination

- Search for metastases in the neck (Virchow's node), abdomen and pelvis.

# Investigations

- Double-contrast barium swallow.
- Upper GI endoscopy (biopsy or brush cytology).
- Endoscopic ultrasound (most precise staging investigation of tumour's depth, but not for nodal status).
- CT or MRI of thorax and abdomen.

- Preliminary studies have suggested that fluoro-2-deoxy-D-glucose positron emission tomography (FDG-PET) can detect otherwise radiographically occult distant metastatic disease.
- Other investigations include:
  - FBC
  - liver function tests (LFTs)
  - CXR
  - bronchoscopy
  - abdominal USS.

# Treatment

- Oesophageal resection:
  - is indicated for operable tumours (40% of all cases)
  - requires peri-operative intensive-care facilities and careful patient selection
  - pre-operative chemotherapy and radiation may be required to downstage advanced tumours to render them operable
  - a proximal margin of 10 cm is preferable
  - should be combined with removal of regional lymph nodes in juxtaposition
  - the Ivor–Lewis operation is suitable for tumours of the middle and lower thirds. The operation usually requires a laparotomy and a thoracotomy. The stomach is pulled through for anastomosis with the proximal oesophagus and a pyloroplasty is performed
  - for tumours of the upper third, McKeown's procedure (laparotomy, right thoracotomy and left neck incision) or a sternotomy approach is used. A stomach pull-through or a jejunal Roux-en-Y can be performed. In some cases, laryngectomy, tracheostomy, pharyngectomy and/or total oesophagectomy may be required
  - thoracoscopic dissection of the oesophagus has recently been developed
  - surgery also has a palliative role (surgical bypass).
- Radiotherapy:
  - response rate is 35%

- complete eradication rate is 5%
  - side-effects include strictures, cardiac and pulmonary damage, bleeding and malignant oesophago-tracheo-bronchial fistula formation.
- Intubation:
  - is indicated for advanced and non-resectable tumours and for unfit patients
  - pulsion or traction technique may be used
  - the funnel of the tube sits proximal to the tumour
  - self-expanding metal stents have been used recently with good results
  - the risk of perforation is 10%
  - intubation is contraindicated in cervical lesions.
- Laser therapy:
  - Nd:YAG laser therapy provides temporary palliation.
- Chemotherapy:
  - there is increasing evidence that chemotherapy (e.g. 5-FU and cisplatin) is effective in oesophageal cancer. Tumour regression occurs in 60% of cases.

# Prognosis

- The 5-year survival rate is 18% for surgical resection.
- Survival rates have been improving due to increased surgical expertise, careful patient selection, use of a multi-modality approach, and earlier detection.

# 13 Gastric cancer

## Epidemiology

- The incidence is 23 per 100 000 per year (declining worldwide).
- It accounts for 6% of all cancer deaths.
- The peak incidence is in the age range 50–70 years.
- The male:female ratio is 2:1.
- The highest incidence is in Japan.
- Pre-malignant changes include chronic atrophic gastritis, intestinal metaplasia and dysplasia.
- Risk factors include *Helicobacter pylori* infection, blood group A, high intake of salt and salt-cured meats, vitamin deficiency (vitamins A, C and E), high intake of nitrates and selenium deficiency.
- Various genetic alterations have been linked to gastric cancer (e.g. p53, C-myc and C-erb B2).

## Pathology

- The lesion may be polypoid, ulcerative, diffuse or ulcerative/diffuse.
- Around 35% of lesions arise in the proximal third.

## Staging

- TNM system (1997 edition).
- The regional lymph nodes include the perigastric nodes, the nodes along the left gastric common hepatic, splenic and coeliac arteries, and the nodes in the hepatoduodenal ligaments.
- N0: no regional node involvement.

- N1: metastasis in 1–6 regional nodes.
- N2: metastasis in 7–15 regional nodes.
- N3: metastasis in more than 15 regional nodes.

# Clinical features

- Dysphagia.
- Vomiting.
- Abdominal pain (50% of cases).
- Epigastric mass (20%).
- Microcytic anaemia.
- Weight loss and cachexia.
- Other features include:
  - Krukenberg's tumour
  - venous thrombosis
  - left supraclavicular lymphadenopathy.

# Investigations

- FBC, serum biochemistry.
- Upper GI endoscopy (and biopsy) and barium meal.
- CT or MRI and/or USS for staging.

# Treatment

- Gastrectomy.
  - This is possible in 65% of cases.
  - Access is through a transverse subcostal incision, vertical midline incision or Ivor–Lewis approach.
  - It entails sufficient resection margins, omentectomy and lymphadenectomy.
  - D1 resection is indicated for pT1 tumours and D2 (extended lymph-node dissection) resection for tumours with serosal involvement. The pancreas and spleen should be preserved if possible.

- There is no evidence that D2 resection improves survival in early gastric cancer, but it may have benefit in tumours > T3.
- For proximal tumours, oesophageal resection may be required in order to achieve a 10 cm proximal margin.
- Billroth II reconstruction is indicated for distal tumours.
- Radical total gastrectomy and oesophago-jejunostomy (Roux-en-Y) are indicated for extensive tumours.
- Gastrectomy for early disease can be performed laparoscopically. Randomised controlled trials comparing laparoscopic gastrectomy with the open approach are required.

- Adjuvant chemotherapy (5-FU plus leucovorin) is considered if more than three nodes are involved.
- Post-operative chemoradiation seems to improve the survival of patients with chemosensitive locally advanced disease.
- Radiotherapy may be given pre-, intra- or post-operatively. Some tumours are rendered operable by neoadjuvant chemotherapy.
- Chemotherapy (5-FU, mitomycin C and adriamycin) may be given in cases of advanced disease.
- Palliative procedures include gastroenterostomy (ante-colic), intubation, dilatation and laser treatment.

# Prognosis

- The 5-year survival rate is 80% for stage IA (T1N0M0) and 10% for stage IV (T4N1–3M0T1–3N3M0 and TanyNanyM1).

# 14

# Gastrointestinal lymphoma (GIL)

## Epidemiology

- This represents 5% of all GI malignancies and 10% of extra-nodal non-Hodgkin's lymphoma.
- It is essential to distinguish between primary GIL and secondary involvement of the GI tract.
- The peak incidence occurs in the age range 50–70 years.
- The male:female ratio is 2:1.
- The incidence of anorectal lymphoma is rising.
- The stomach is the commonest site for GIL (35–79% of cases).

## Aetiology

- Malignant transformation of mucosa-associated lymphatic tissue (MALT) seems to be important in pathogenesis.
- Predisposing factors include:
  - atrophic gastritis (*Helicobacter pylori*)
  - α-chain disease
  - coeliac disease
  - dermatitis herpetiformis
  - Crohn's disease
  - autoimmune disorders
  - immunodeficiency syndromes, including AIDS.

# Pathology

- Stage I: tumour confined to GI organs.
- Stage II: tumour with intra-abdominal lymph node involvement.
- Stage III: extra-abdominal nodes or other organs involved.
- Stage IV: disseminated disease.

There are three main types:

- western lymphoma (non-Hodgkin's B-cell lymphoma)
- primary lymphoma associated with coeliac disease (T-cell lymphoma)
- Mediterranean lymphoma associated with α-chain disease.

# Clinical features

- Symptoms include:
  - abdominal pain
  - nausea
  - vomiting
  - weight loss
  - fatigue.
- Physical examination may reveal an abdominal mass (35% of cases) and anaemia.
- Symptoms and signs of obstruction, perforation or haemorrhage.

# Investigations

- FBC, serum U&Es and LFTs.
- CXR (with thoracic CT).
- Abdominal ultrasonography.
- Abdomino-pelvic CT.
- Gastrointestinal endoscopy (with biopsy).
- Endosonography.
- Barium studies of the GI tract.
- Faecal occult blood testing.

- Southern blot DNA hybridisation of fresh biopsy specimens.
- Laparotomy/laparoscopy.

# Management

- Treatment depends upon the site, stage and histological subtype.
  - Stage I and II disease is treated by resection of the involved segment (e.g. subtotal gastrectomy, right hemicolectomy, etc.) with the regional lymph nodes. Post-operative radiotherapy (25 Gy to the whole abdomen with a boost of 15 Gy to the tumour region) and adjuvant chemotherapy with cyclophosphamide, doxorubicin, vincristine and prednisolone (CHOP) are recommended if the lesion is high grade and/or the margins of the resection specimens are involved in the disease.
  - Stage III and IV disease is treated by chemotherapy (cyclophosphamide, doxorubicin hydrochloride, oncovin and prednisolone (CHOP)) and radiotherapy, with a 50% response rate. Surgical intervention is reserved for complications such as obstruction, haemorrhage and perforation.

# Prognosis

- The 5-year survival rate for stages I and II is 70% for completely resected tumours and 40% for incompletely resected lesions.
- The 5-year survival rate for stages III and IV is 20%.

# 15 Small bowel carcinoma

## Epidemiology

- This accounts for 40% of all small bowel malignancies. The latter account for 5% of all GI malignancies.
- The male:female ratio is 2:1.
- The average age at presentation is 50 years.
- The duodenum and proximal jejunum are the commonest sites.

## Aetiology

- Predisposing factors include Crohn's disease, coeliac disease, Peutz–Jegher's syndrome, adenomatous polyps and polyposis syndromes.

## Clinical features

- Symptoms include:
  - diarrhoea
  - anaemia
  - abdominal pain
  - nausea
  - vomiting
  - haemorrhage
  - perforation
  - intermittent jaundice (duodenal lesions)
  - anorexia
  - weight loss.

- Signs include:
  - anaemia
  - abdominal mass
  - jaundice
  - signs of obstruction or perforation.

# Investigations

- FBC, serum U&Es, LFTs, faecal occult blood testing.
- Barium meal and follow-through series reveal tumour in 50% of cases.
- GI endoscopy and biopsy.
- CXR.
- Abdominal USS and/or CT.
- Laparoscopy/laparotomy.

# Management

- Wide surgical resection including the regional lymph nodes is the mainstay of management.
- Whipple's operation may be necessary for duodenal lesions.
- Surgical palliation may involve intestinal resection or bypass.
- Radiotherapy and chemotherapy play little role in treatment.
- The role of nitrosoureas and 5-FU is currently being investigated.

# Prognosis

- The lesions are usually advanced at the time of diagnosis.
- The incidence of metastases is approximately 70% at the time of laparotomy.
- The 5-year survival rate is 35% for duodenal lesions and 20% for lesions elsewhere.

*Note:* Other primary malignancies of the small bowel include:

- carcinoids (30%)
- lymphoma (18%)
- sarcoma (15%).

# 16 Colorectal carcinoma

## Epidemiology

- The incidence ranges from 0.4 per 100 000 per year (in Nigeria) to 32.3 per 100 000 per year (in the USA).

## Aetiology

- Risk factors include:
  - familial polyposis coli (FPC)
  - Lynch syndrome I and II
  - high intake of dietary fat
  - low intake of dietary fibre
  - obesity
  - high alcohol intake
  - bile acids
  - tobacco smoking
  - asbestos
  - ulcerative colitis
  - Crohn's disease
  - family history of colorectal cancer
  - previous history of colorectal polyps or cancer
  - ureterosigmoidostomy.
- The adenoma–carcinoma sequence is important in colorectal carcinogenesis.
- Genetic alterations in growth suppressor genes (p53 and BRCA-1) and oncogenes (K-ras) cause tissue change from normal epithelium to adenoma and then carcinoma.
- COX-2 inhibitors seem to reduce the risk.

# Screening

- Patients with colorectal cancer, polyps, ulcerative colitis and a family history of polyposis syndromes should be screened with colonoscopy.
- Other screening methods include barium enema, flexible sigmoidoscopy and faecal occult blood (FOB) testing.

# Pathology

- Around 98% of cancers are adenocarcinomas. The tumour is confined to the mucosal and sub-mucosal layers in Dukes' A, has penetrated the bowel wall (muscularis mucosa) in Dukes' B, and there is regional lymph node involvement in Dukes' C. There are distant metastases in Dukes' D.
- The incidence of lymph node metastasis depends upon the tumour grade and the presence of p53 oncogenes.

# Clinical features

- Large bowel obstruction (more likely with left-sided lesions).
- Perforation and peritonitis.
- Altered bowel habits.
- Rectal bleeding.
- Microcytic anaemia (more likely with right-sided lesions).
- Small bowel obstruction (e.g. caecal carcinoma).
- Abdominal mass.
- Symptoms and signs of metastasis (e.g. hepatomegaly and ascites).

# Investigations

- Proctosigmoidoscopy.
- FBC.
- LFTs.

- Serum carcino-embryonic antigen (CEA).
- Barium enema.
- Colonoscopy.
- Abdominal ultrasonography (including liver).
- Endoscopic biopsy.
- Abdomino-pelvic CT.
- Other investigations include:
  - IVU for suspected ureter involvement
  - bone scan
  - CXR and brain CT for suspected metastases.

# Treatment

- Surgical excision is the main treatment. Right hemicolectomy, transverse colectomy, left hemicolectomy, sigmoid colectomy, anterior and abdominoperineal excision of the rectum may be performed.
  - The amount of large bowel removed depends upon the aetiology, arterial blood supply, grade of differentiation, quality of the anal sphincters and the patient's age and fitness.
  - A permanent stoma is necessary if the tumour invades the anal sphincters, if the tumour is located within 5 cm of the dentate line and is poorly differentiated or if the anal sphincters are weak and uncontrollable and incontinence is likely.
  - The distal clearance margin should be $\geq 2$ cm for well-differentiated tumours and $\geq 5$ cm for poorly differentiated tumours.
  - Total excision of the mesorectum reduces the incidence of local recurrence of rectal cancer and prolongs survival.
  - Radiotherapy administered pre-operatively or post-operatively improves disease-free survival in patients with rectal carcinoma.
  - A loop ileostomy may be performed to protect a low anastomosis.
  - Subtotal colectomy and ileo-rectal anastomosis is indicated in cases of FPC, Lynch syndrome and younger patients with left-sided obstruction.

- A colonic pouch–anal anastomosis may be performed for very low rectal tumours.
- The role of laparoscopic surgery and sentinel-node biopsy in the surgical treatment of colorectal cancer is currently under investigation.
- Adjuvant chemotherapy (5-FU plus folinic acid infusion) for 6 months is indicated for stage II rectal cancer and stage III colonic and rectal carcinoma.
- The addition of oxaliplatin or capecitabine to 5-FU and folinic acid infusion seems to improve survival in patients with metastatic disease.
- Biological therapy with monoclonal antibodies against vascular endothelial growth factor (bevacizumab) or epidermal growth factor (cetuximab) seems to be effective in the treatment of metastatic disease.
- Radiotherapy is indicated in rectal cancer (Dukes' B and C). It may be given post-operatively or pre-operatively. It is also useful for inoperable or recurrent cancers.
- Management of locally advanced disease.
  - *En bloc* surgical excision is the mainstay of management.
  - Ureter involvement can be managed with ureteroureterostomy, Boari flap reconstruction, ileal conduit, ureterostomy, spout colostomy diversion or nephrostomy.
  - For rectal cancer, radiotherapy (with or without chemotherapy) may be given pre-operatively to shrink tumours or post-operatively for involved margins.
  - Chemotherapy in the form of systemic 5-FU/folinic acid infusion should be given to fit patients. Recent evidence suggests that regimens containing irinotecan, oxaliplatin and/or bevacizumab (monoclonal antibody directed against vascular endothelial growth factor) are more effective than standard 5-FU plus folinic acid infusion in patients with advanced colorectal cancer.
- Management of liver metastases.
  - Hepatic resection is possible in 25% of cases, and the 5-year survival rate is 20% after surgery. Post-operative regional (intra-arterial/portal) chemotherapy reduces the relapse rate.

- Systemic 5-FU and folinic acid may be given for inoperable liver metastases, with a 30% response rate. Raltitrexed is effective in the palliation of metastatic disease.
- Management of other metastases.
  - Radiotherapy is indicated for bony metastases.
  - Radiotherapy and corticosteroids are indicated for brain metastases.
- Management of local recurrence.
  - Clinical local recurrence occurs in around 10% of cases.
  - Around 70% of patients with local recurrence have distant metastases.
  - Treatment modalities include surgical excision, endoluminal excision (using diathermy or laser) and/or radiotherapy.

# Prognosis

- The 5-year survival rate is 90% for Dukes' A, 55% for Dukes' B, 30% for Dukes' C and 15% for Dukes' D.

# Follow-up

- History and examination (including rigid sigmoidoscopy) are performed every 3 months for the first 3 years and then every 6 months thereafter.
- Serum CEA may be measured regularly.
- Colonoscopic surveillance should be undertaken every 4 years for patients presenting with a single cancer and every 2 years for those presenting with multiple cancers.

# 17 Anal cancer

## Epidemiology

- The incidence ranges from 0.2 per 100 000 per year (in the Philippines) to 3.6 per 100 000 per year (in Switzerland).
- The incidence is increasing worldwide.

## Aetiology

- Risk factors include:
  - receptive anal intercourse
  - human papilloma virus (HPV) types 16, 18, 31 and 33
  - herpes simplex virus type II
  - *Chlamydia* and HIV infection.

## Pathology

- Around 80% of lesions are epidermoid, and the remainder consist of melanoma and adenocarcinoma.
- Local spread tends to occur in the cephalad direction.
- Nodal spread to perirectal, inguinal and lateral pelvic nodes may occur.

## Clinical features

- Pain and bleeding in 50% of cases.
- Anal mass/ulcer, faecal incontinence and/or ano-vaginal fistula.
- Inguinal lymphadenopathy in 30% of cases (metastases are confirmed in only 50% of such cases).
- Hepatomegaly (uncommon).

# Investigations

- Proctoscopy and biopsy.
- Examination under anaesthetic (EUA) and biopsy.
- Endo-anal USS.
- CT or MRI.

# Treatment

- Combined radiotherapy (50 Gy) and chemotherapy (5-FU and mitomycin C) is the mainstay of management (Nigro's regimen).
- Surgical treatment is indicated for failure of primary non-surgical therapy (residual tumour, radionecrosis, fistulae and local recurrence), for small lesions at the anal margin and for inguinal recurrence after radiotherapy.
- Surgical procedures include abdominoperineal resection, de-functioning colostomy, excision of peri-anal lesions and inguinal node dissection.
- Adenocarcinoma is usually treated with abdominoperineal resection, and melanoma is treated with more conservative surgery due to the poor prognosis.

# Prognosis

- The overall 5-year survival rate for epidermoid carcinoma is 58%. The local control rate with radiotherapy and chemotherapy is 90%.

# 18 Gall bladder cancer

## Epidemiology

- Gall bladder cancer is found incidentally in 2% of all gall bladders excised for gallstones.
- The peak incidence occurs in the age range 60–80 years.
- The male:female ratio is 2:5.

## Aetiology

- It is associated with gallstones in 75% of cases.
- Carcinogens, including nitrosamines and methylcholanthrene.
- A higher incidence is reported among those working in the rubber industry and typhoid carriers.

## Pathology

- The histological subtypes include adenocarcinoma (85%), squamous-cell carcinoma (3%) and undifferentiated (7%).
- The tumour tends to invade locally.
- Spread may occur via the intraductal lymphatic or vascular routes.
- The lesion appears macroscopically as a nodule, polypoid mass or focal/diffuse thickening.

# Clinical features

- Incidental finding in a cholecystectomy specimen.
- Pain (80% of cases), nausea and vomiting (50%), weight loss (40%), jaundice (40%), abdominal distension (30%), pruritus (15%) and melaena (3%).
- Hepatomegaly (40%), mass in the right hypochondrium (40%) and upper abdominal tenderness (40%).

# Investigations

- FBC and LFTs.
- Ultrasound, CT and/or MRI.
- Cholangiography (ERCP/PTC).

# Nevin's staging

- Stage I: mucosa only.
- Stage II: mucosa and muscularis.
- Stage III: transmural.
- Stage IV: transmural and cystic lymph node.
- Stage V: liver invasion/distant metastases.

# Treatment

- Simple open cholecystectomy for stages I and II.
- Radical cholecystectomy, including adjacent liver resection and regional lymph node dissection, for stages III and IV. Pancreaticoduodenectomy is performed in selected cases. Radical surgery may be performed for stage V in fit patients.
- Palliative procedures include stenting (endoscopic or percutaneous) and surgical bypass (Roux-en-Y hepatico-jejunostomy).
- Intra-operative radiotherapy for stages III, IV and V.

# Prognosis

- The 5-year survival rate is 60% for stage I, 40% for stage II, 10% for stage III, 7% for stage IV and 1% for stage V.

# 19
# Cholangiocarcinoma

## Epidemiology

- This accounts for 1.5% of all cancers.
- It is more common in the sixth and seventh decades and among males.

## Aetiology

- Risk factors include:
  - gallstones (found in 30% of cases)
  - choledochal cysts
  - Caroli's disease
  - sclerosing cholangitis
  - ulcerative colitis
  - *Clonorchis sinesis* infestation (liver fluke)
  - *Opsithorchis viverrini* infestation
  - thorium dioxide and drugs (OCP and methyldopa).

## Pathology

- The common bile duct (CBD) is the commonest location (40% of cases), followed by the common hepatic duct (32%), hepatic duct bifurcation (20%) and cystic duct (5%).
- Adenocarcinoma is the commonest type (97%).
- The tumour may be peripheral (type I), hilar (type II), middle third extrahepatic (type III) or distal extrahepatic (type IV).

# Clinical features

- Jaundice is the commonest presentation (95%).
- Abdominal pain.
- Hepatomegaly.
- Pruritus.
- Abdominal tenderness.
- Ascites.
- Abnormal LFTs.

# Investigations

- LFTs.
- Ultrasound, CT and/or MRI scan.
- Cholangiography (ERCP and/or PTC).
- Angiography or Doppler study to assess resectability.

# Treatment and prognosis

- Resectable tumours of the distal third of the CBD are treated with radical pancreaticoduodenectomy (Whipple's procedure). The 5-year survival rate is 50%.
- The resectable tumours of the middle third are treated with excision (1 cm clear margin) and biliary–intestinal anastomosis (hepatico-jejunostomy). The 5-year survival rate is 50%.
- For proximal hilar tumours, 'attempt-at-cure' surgery has been proposed. The surgery involves local excision alone for type I, local excision and partial hepatectomy for types II and III, or orthoptic liver transplantation (OLT) for type IV. The 3-year survival rate is 30%. The resectability rate is 20% (compared with 65% for tumours of the middle and distal thirds of the CBD).
- Partial hepatectomy or OLT is indicated for peripheral cholangiocarcinoma. The 3-year survival rate is 50%.

- Palliative procedures for unresectable tumours or unfit patients include stent placement (endoscopic or percutaneous trans-hepatic) and surgical biliary–intestinal anastomosis. Self-expandable stainless steel endoprostheses are preferable for palliation. The median survival is 8 months.
- With regard to adjuvant therapy, chemotherapy and radio-therapy have no established role in management as yet.

# 20 Hepatocellular carcinoma (HCC)

## Epidemiology

- This is the commonest primary cancer of the liver.
- The male:female ratio is 3:2.
- The peak incidence occurs in the age range 40–60 years.

## Aetiology

- Risk factors include:
  - aflatoxin and algal toxins
  - hepatic cirrhosis
  - viral hepatitis (B and C)
  - haemochromatosis
  - $\alpha_1$-antitrypsin deficiency
  - tobacco smoking
  - oestrogenic steroids
  - autoimmune chronic hepatitis
  - primary biliary cirrhosis
  - Wilson's disease.

## Pathology

- The tumour type may be:
  - diffuse
  - single
  - encapsulated
  - fibrolamellar.

# Clinical features

- Pain:
  - epigastric
  - right hypochondrium
  - back.
- Anorexia.
- Dyspnoea (lung metastases/pleural effusion).
- Ascites.
- Hepatomegaly.
- Bleeding.
- Oesophageal varices.
- Obstructive jaundice.
- Bony metastases.
- Arterial murmur over the tumour.
- Paraneoplastic symptoms include:
  - fever
  - hypoglycaemia
  - hypercalcaemia
  - polycythaemia.

# Investigations

- FBC, serum biochemistry and clotting screen.
- Serum α-fetoprotein (AFP) is a useful marker.
- Hepatitis screen (for hepatitis B and C).
- Abdominal (sunburst calcification) and chest X-ray.
- CT scan and ultrasound scan, angiography, Doppler flow studies and/or portal venography.
- FNAC or core biopsy under radiological guidance. Biopsy should be avoided in patients coming for resection or transplantation, in order to prevent tumour spread along the needle track.

# Treatment

- Peripheral wedge resection of small superficial carcinomas.

- Hepatic segmental resection is the mainstay of curative treatment. Patients with multi-centric tumours, severe liver impairment, ascites and distant metastases are excluded.
- Orthoptic liver transplantation should be offered to carefully selected patients without dissemination who are not suitable for segmental resection.
- Intra-arterial chemotherapy. The results of systemic chemotherapy remain disappointing.
- Interferon-$\alpha$ is effective, especially in reducing the recurrence rate.
- Arterial embolisation is particularly effective in the management of ruptured HCC.
  - It is performed percutaneously using Gelfoam, Ivalon, steel coils or starch microspheres.
  - Post-embolisation syndrome consists of pyrexia, pain, nausea and worsening LFTs.
  - Arterial embolisation is contraindicated in the presence of portal vein thrombosis.
- Percutaneous ethanol injection causes complete necrosis in more than 90% of small tumours (< 3 cm in diameter).
- Radiotherapy may be given in the form of external beam radiation, percutaneous injection of radioactive material or transcatheter injection of $[^{131}I]$-lipiodol.
- The role of tamoxifen is questionable.

# Prognosis

- The 3-year survival rate for resection is 40%.
- The 3-year survival rate for transplantation is 25%.
- The 1-year survival rate for untreated patients is 20%.

# 21 Carcinoma of the pancreas

## Epidemiology

- The incidence ranges from 2 to 15 per 100 000 per year depending upon geographical location. The incidence is increasing.
- The female:male ratio is 3:1.
- The peak incidence is in the age range 60–80 years.

## Aetiology

- Pancreatic cancer is associated with:
  - cigarette smoking (2.5-fold increase in risk)
  - high intake of animal fats and coffee
  - pancreatitis (hereditary or chronic)
  - ataxia telangiectasia.

## Pathology

- The tumour type may be:
  - ductal (82%)
  - giant cell (6%)
  - adenosquamous (4%)
  - mucinous adenocarcinoma (2%)
  - mucinous cystadenocarcinoma (1%)
  - acinar-cell carcinoma (1%).

# Clinical features

- Jaundice (pancreatic head tumours).
- Pain.
- Weight loss.
- Pancreatitis.
- Upper GI haemorrhage.
- Thromboembolic disease.
- Cholangitis.
- Psychiatric disturbance.
- Thrombophlebitis.
- Migraine.
- Upper abdominal mass.
- Constipation.
- Bloating.
- Diarrhoea.
- Fatigue.
- Palpable gall bladder.
- Splenomegaly.
- Hepatomegaly.
- Diabetes mellitus.

# Investigations

- FBC, serum U&Es, LFTs, clotting screen, ultrasonography, ERCP and CT scanning.
- Brush cytology, FNAC or core biopsy under radiological guidance.
- The staging investigations include:
  - colour flow Doppler ultrasonography
  - spiral CT scanning
  - angiography
  - laparoscopy
  - endoscopic ultrasonography
  - laparotomy.

# Treatment

- Correction of clotting and electrolyte abnormalities.
- Surgical resection.
  - This is indicated for small tumours (< 3 cm in diameter) and favourable histological types in the absence of distant metastases.
  - It is possible in 8–25% of patients.
  - Whipple's operation is indicated for tumours of the head, and distal pancreatectomy for tumours of the body and tail. More radical resection does not improve survival.
  - Whipple's operation entails proximal pancreatectomy, gastroduodenal resection, cholecystectomy, pancreatico-jejunostomy, choledochojejunostomy and gastrojejunostomy.
  - The post-operative mortality rate should be less than 5%.
  - The post-operative morbidity rate remains high (30–50%).
- Palliative surgery.
  - Choledochoduodenostomy and retrocolic gastrojejunostomy.
  - Endoscopic stent placement (self-expanding metal-mesh stents are preferable).
  - There is no difference in survival between surgical bypass and stenting.
- Radiotherapy.
  - This may be given adjuvantly after resection.
  - Radiotherapy and 5-FU increase the survival rate in non-resectable tumours.
- Chemotherapy.
  - 5-FU and mitomycin seem to be effective agents. The objective response rate is 20%.
- Coeliac plexus block can be used for pain palliation.
- Biological therapy (e.g. angiogenesis inhibitors and immunotherapy) is likely to play a part in the treatment of this disease.

# Prognosis

- The median survival after surgical resection is 18 months (it is longer for mucinous adenocarcinoma).
- The average survival after palliation is 5.4 months.
- The average 5-year survival rate is 2–5%.

# 22 Multiple endocrine neoplasia (MEN) syndromes

- MEN I:
  - autosomal dominant inheritance
  - involves pituitary, islet cells of pancreas and parathyroid glands
  - thyroid adenomas, carcinoids, adrenal adenomas, thymomas and ovarian tumours are associated with MEN I.
- MEN IIa:
  - autosomal dominant inheritance
  - includes medullary thyroid carcinoma (MTC), phaeo-chromocytoma and parathyroid adenoma or hyperplasia.
- MEN IIb:
  - autosomal dominant or sporadic
  - includes phaeochromocytoma, MTC, submucosal neuromas, ganglioneuromas and marfanoid habitus.

# 23 Insulinoma

## Pathology

- Originates in the β-cells of the pancreatic islets.
- Around 90% of insulinomas are small single adenomas.
- Insulinomas associated with MEN I are multiple in 75% of cases.
- Around 10% of insulinomas are malignant.

## Clinical features

- The clinical picture is defined by Whipple's triad:
  - symptoms and signs of hypoglycaemia occurring during fasting or exercise
  - at the time of symptoms, the blood glucose level is below 60 mg/dl
  - the symptoms are reversed by glucose administration.

## Investigations

- Serum insulin:glucose ratio, which usually exceeds 1 in insulinoma patients.
- Localisation using selective venous sampling, angiography, CT and/or MRI.
- Intra-operative USS.
- Provocative tests.

# Treatment

- Small benign lesions can be enucleated.
- Malignant lesions are treated by pancreatic resection (distal pancreatectomy or Whipple's operation). Stropozotocin is an effective chemotherapeutic agent.

# Prognosis

- The median survival for malignant tumours is 5 years after curative resection.
- The median disease-free survival falls to 4 years after palliative resection.

# 24 Gastrinoma

## Pathology

- A non-β-islet-cell tumour of the pancreas is the commonest cause.
- Around 60% of tumours are malignant.
- Around 65% of cases occur in the pancreas and 35% in the duodenum.
- Gastrinoma is associated with MEN I.

## Clinical features

- Causes hypergastrinaemia and hypersecretion of gastric acid (atypical peptic ulceration, Zollinger–Ellison syndrome).

## Investigations

- Serum gastrin and gastric acid output.
- Secretin test.
- Localisation with arteriography, upper gastrointestinal series, CT, selective venous sampling and/or MRI.

## Treatment

- Surgical resection of well-localised tumours. Only 20% of tumours are resectable.
- Medical treatment with omeprazole, lansoprazole, somatostatin analogues and/or streptozotocin.
- Total gastrectomy is a recognised treatment modality.

# 25 Malignant phaeochromocytoma

## Pathology

- Arises from the neural crest-derived chromaffin tissue.
- Accounts for approximately 7% of phaeochromocytomas.
- Around 90% of tumours are found in the adrenal medulla.
- Secretes excess amounts of adrenaline and noradrenaline.

## Clinical features

- Usually presents with general symptoms such as hypertension, palpitations, headache, anxiety, nausea and vomiting, and local symptoms depending upon location.

## Investigations

- Diagnosis is based on elevated serum and urinary catecholamines (VMA, adrenaline and noradrenaline).
- Neuron-specific enolase is a useful marker.
- Localisation using $[^{131}I]$-MIBG (metiodobenzylguanidine) scan (95% accuracy), CT and/or MRI.
- Vena cava sampling is occasionally performed.

# Treatment

- Pre-operative preparation includes α-blockade (3 weeks of phenoxybenzamine), $\beta_1$-blockade and correction of vascular volume.
- Surgical removal of tumour.
- Embolisation.
- α- and β-blockers for symptom control.
- [$^{131}$I]-MIBG scan and chemotherapy (cyclophosphamide, vincristine and dacarbazine).

# Prognosis

- The 5-year survival rate is 40%.

# 26 Adrenocortical malignancy

## Epidemiology

- The incidence is 0.1 per 100 000 per year.
- Women are more commonly affected.
- The peak incidence occurs during the fourth decade.

## Pathology

- Tumours may be non-functioning (compressing and invading surrounding structures) or functioning, causing Cushing's syndrome (50%), virilisation (30%), feminisation (12%) or Conn's syndrome (very rare).
- Around 40% of patients have metastases at presentation.

## Investigations

- Biochemical measurement (serum cortisol, ACTH, steroid suppression tests, etc.).
- CT, USS, MRI, IVU, angiography and/or selective venous sampling.
- CT-guided biopsy.

## Treatment

- Adrenalectomy (lateral or anterior approach).

- Chemotherapy (mitotane, streptozotocin, 5-FU, doxorubicin and/or cisplatin).

# Prognosis

- The 5-year survival rate is 20%.

# 27 Carcinoid tumours

## Epidemiology

- Carcinoid tumours arise from amine precursor uptake decarboxylase (APUD) cells and secrete serotonin.
- The incidence is 1.5 per 100 000 per year.

## Pathology

- Around 75% of the tumours occur in the mid-gut with 45% in the appendix.

## Clinical features

- Carcinoids present with local symptoms (appendicitis or bowel obstruction) or symptoms of the carcinoid syndrome (found in 9% of cases).
- Right cardiac complications occur in 50% of cases.

## Investigations

- The investigation of choice is 24-hourly urinary 5-hydroxyindole acetic acid (5-HIAA) measurement.
- Barium studies, colonoscopy, CT, MRI, USS and/or laparoscopy.

# Management

- Surgery.
  - For non-metastatic primary tumours or obstructive intestinal lesions.
  - Appendix: appendicectomy for lesions < 2 cm in diameter and right hemicolectomy for lesions > 2 cm in diameter.
  - Stomach and duodenum: local excision for tumours < 1 cm in diameter.
  - Small bowel: small bowel resection with mesentery.
  - Rectum: local excision if lesion is < 2 cm in diameter and excision of rectum if lesion is > 2 cm in diameter.
  - Solitary metastasis in liver can be treated by hepatic resection.
- Somatostatin analogs such as octreotide and lanreotide for the carcinoid syndrome.
- Chemotherapy.
  - The role is not clearly defined.
  - It may be given for metastatic disease or as an adjuvant to surgery and/or radiotherapy.
  - The response rate is 33%. No survival benefit has been demonstrated.
  - 5-FU, streptozotocin, doxorubicin and cyclophosphamide are usually used.
- Embolisation for hepatic metastases.
- Interferons.
- Other drugs include histamine antagonists and 5-HT antagonists.
- Other treatments:
  - brachytherapy
  - photodynamic therapy
  - endoscopic mucosectomy
  - surgical bypass (Kirschner operation)
  - electrocoagulation
  - ethanol injection
  - radionuclide ablation.

# Prognosis

- The 5-year survival rate is 5%.

# 28 Thyroid cancer

## Epidemiology

- The incidence is 3.1 per 100 000 per year.
- The female:male ratio is 2.5:1.

## Aetiology

- Radiation (accounts for 10% of cases).
- Genetic factors (medullary thyroid carcinoma, MTC).
- Pre-existing benign conditions (e.g. Hashimoto's thyroiditis, multinodular and endemic goitres).

## Pathology

- Papillary tumours:
    - account for 70% of cases
    - are usually low grade
    - the incidence of multifocal and bilateral disease is 80%
    - the regional lymph nodes are involved in 50% of cases.
- Follicular tumours:
    - account for 16% of cases
    - lymph-node metastases occur in 5% of cases
    - vascular invasion is a poor prognostic indicator
    - Hürthle-cell carcinoma is a cytological variant of follicular carcinoma.
- Medullary tumours:
    - account for 6% of cases
    - arise in parafollicular C-cells
    - there is an association with MEN syndrome (type IIa)

- calcitonin is a useful serum marker
- the tumours may secrete ACTH and prostaglandins.
- Anaplastic carcinoma:
  - accounts for 7% of cases
  - occurs predominantly in the elderly and carries a poor prognosis.
- Lymphoma:
  - accounts for 1% of thyroid tumours
  - is usually of the non-Hodgkin's type
  - poor prognostic indicators include spread beyond the cervical nodes, necrosis and vascular invasion.

# Clinical presentation

- Incidental pathological findings in a thyroidectomy specimen excised for benign disease.
- Discrete thyroid nodule. Around 5% of all solitary nodules are malignant.
- Recently enlarging, multinodular goitre.
- Cervical lymphadenopathy.
- Neck mass with pressure symptoms.
- Voice change.
- Distant metastases.

# Investigations

- Fine-needle aspiration cytology. This is the most useful investigation.
- Thyroid function tests.
- Ultrasonography.
- Core biopsy may be considered in some cases.
- CXR.
- CT and MRI may be useful for assessing the extent of disease.
- Radioactive iodine scan following total thyroidectomy.
- Serum calcitonin for medullary tumours.
- Serum thyroglobulin and its antibodies to screen for recurrence after complete thyroidectomy.

# Management

- Total thyroidectomy and removal of involved lymph nodes. The recurrent laryngeal nerve should be identified and preserved. Attempts should also be made to preserve the parathyroids. Unilateral lobectomy is adequate for solitary tumours less than 1 cm in diameter. The sentinel-node biopsy may be used to assess the nodal status.
- Thyroxine is used to suppress thyroid-stimulating hormone (TSH) activity.
- Radioactive iodine ($[^{131}I]$) is used for follicular carcinoma, advanced papillary carcinoma (stages II to IV) and metastatic disease.
- External beam radiation is used for inadequately excised papillary, follicular, medullary and Hürthle-cell carcinomas.
- External radiation and chemotherapy are used to control anaplastic carcinoma.
- Lymphoma is treated by radiotherapy. Chemotherapy is indicated if there is retrosternal or distant spread.

# Follow-up

- Physical examination.
- Thyroid function tests.
- Serum thyroglobulin and its antibody.
- Radioactive iodine ($[^{131}I]$) scan.
- Serum calcitonin (medullary carcinoma).

# Prognosis

Prognostic factors include the histological type, the tumour's size and degree of differentiation, nodal spread, distant metastases, multifocality, the patient's age (age above 45 years is a poor prognostic factor) and whether the tumour is genetically determined.

- Papillary carcinoma:
  - low-risk category tumours have a 10-year survival rate of 97%
  - high-risk category tumours have a 10-year survival rate of 85%.
- Follicular carcinoma:
  - low-risk category tumours have a 10-year survival rate of 89%
  - high-risk category tumours have a 10-year survival rate of 73%.
- Medullary carcinoma:
  - the 5- and 10-year survival rates are 69% and 65%, respectively
  - hereditary cases are associated with a worse clinical outcome than sporadic cases.
- Anaplastic carcinoma:
  - the 3-year survival rate is 3%.

# Screening for MTC

- The gene responsible for MTC and MEN II (the RET proto-oncogene) has been localised to chromosome 10q11.2.
- First-degree relatives of patients with MTC should be screened for MTC and other endocrine neoplasms such as parathyroid adenoma and phaeochromocytoma.
- Screening for MTC includes physical examination, serum calcitonin, PTH, VMA, cytogenetics and biopsy.
- Medullary thyroid hyperplasia is a pre-malignant condition and is a recognised indication for prophylactic total thyroidectomy.

# 29 Parathyroid carcinoma

## Epidemiology

- This accounts for 1% of all cases of primary hyperthyroidism.
- It is equally common in men and women.
- It is a rare tumour.

## Pathology

- Histological diagnosis is often difficult.
- Chief cells predominate.
- Flow cytometric analysis of DNA aids the diagnosis.

## Presentation

- Symptoms of hypercalcaemia, including renal stones (56% of cases) and bone involvement (90%).
- Acute pancreatitis (12%).
- Neck mass (45%).

## Investigations

- Serum calcium and parathyroid hormone (levels are higher than in benign disease).
- FNAC.
- Localisation with CT, MRI or thallium–technetium scanning.

# Treatment

- Treatment of hypercalcaemia (with rehydration and bisphosphonates).
- Removal of the tumour en masse with the thyroid lobe, lymph nodes and ipsilateral isthmus.
- The nerve may be sacrificed if it is involved.
- Most patients require oral calcium and vitamin D.

# Prognosis

- Frequent measurement of serum calcium and PTH levels is required during follow-up.
- The 5-year survival rate is 50%.
- The 5-year local recurrence rate is 45%.

# 30 Soft tissue sarcoma (STS)

## Epidemiology

- This accounts for 1% of adult cancers and 15% of paediatric cancers.
- The sex distribution is approximately equal.
- Around 43% of cases arise in the lower extremity, 16% in the upper extremity, 13% in the visceral organs, 12% in the retroperitoneum, 10% in the trunk, 5% in the head and neck and 3% in the chest.

## Aetiology

- The aetiology is unknown in most cases.
- The risk factors include genetic disorders (Li-Fraumeni syndrome, hereditary retinoblastoma, neurofibromatosis and Gardner's syndrome), radiation, lymphoedema, thorium oxide (angio-sarcoma) and vinyl chloride.

## Pathology

- The likelihood of metastasising is greater than 50% for high-grade sarcomas, compared with less than 15% for low-grade sarcomas.
- Immunohistochemical analysis (utilising a panel of antibodies) is used to specify sarcoma type.
- Lymph-node metastases occur in less than 35% of cases.

# Clinical features

- Extremity sarcomas present as a painless mass. The presence of pain indicates a poor prognosis. In general, soft tissue masses which are large in size (> 5 cm in diameter), painful, located deep to superficial fascia and/or increasing rapidly in size should raise the suspicion of sarcoma.
- Retroperitoneal sarcoma patients present with abdominal mass, abdominal pain, neurological symptoms or bowel obstruction.
- Other symptoms include abnormal uterine bleeding (uterine sarcoma), haematuria (bladder sarcoma) and nasal bleeding/obstruction (nasal and paranasal sarcomas).

# Diagnosis

- Core biopsy is more informative than FNAC.
- CT and/or MRI to assess the extent of disease.
- CXR.

# Treatment

- Extremity and trunk. Limb-sparing surgery is an important principle of treatment.
    - Low-grade tumours of the extremity and trunk are treated by wide local resection. External radiotherapy is indicated for large (> 5 cm in diameter) or incompletely excised tumours.
    - High-grade tumours are treated by wide local resection followed by adjuvant radiotherapy (brachytherapy/external radiotherapy). Chemotherapy may be considered for large high-grade sarcomas (> 10 cm in diameter). Lung metastases should be excluded prior to treatment.
- Retroperitoneal and visceral sarcomas are treated by surgical resection. Incompletely excised tumours and large (> 10 cm in diameter) high-grade tumours should be considered for radiotherapy and chemotherapy.

- Gastrointestinal sarcomas may cause bleeding, perforation, ulceration and/or obstruction. These complications require appropriate surgical treatment.
- A minimal 2 cm margin of normal tissue is required for adequate excision.

## Investigations

- Excisional biopsy for superficial tumours < 3 cm in diameter.
- Incisional biopsy or core biopsy (which has limitations) for large and deeply seated tumours.
- LFTs, serum U&Es and FBC.
- MRI scan (superior to CT).
- CXR.
- Thoracic CT if CXR suggests the presence of metastases.
- USS or CT of liver.

## Notes

- Pulmonary metastases can be excised surgically so long as there is good local control of the primary tumour and there is no evidence of extrapulmonary metastases. The 5-year survival rate is 26% following resection.
- Metastatic sarcoma can be treated by chemotherapy (e.g. doxorubicin and ifosfamide), with response rates approaching 35%.
- Local recurrence is treated by surgical excision and radiotherapy.

## Follow-up

- Patients with high-grade tumours of the extremity and trunk should be examined and have a CXR every 3 months for the first 3 years, twice a year for the next 2 years and annually thereafter. A thoracic CT may be performed.

- Patients with visceral and retroperitoneal sarcomas should also have an abdominal CT during follow-up.

# Prognosis

- Depends upon the size, grade and site of the tumour, the adequacy of excision and the histopathological type.
- The 5-year survival rate is 25% for retroperitoneal sarcoma and 80% for extremity sarcoma.

# 31 Kaposi's sarcoma

## Epidemiology

- Kaposi's sarcoma (KS) is relatively common among elderly men (over 50 years) of Mediterranean origin, Ashkenasi Jews and individuals infected with herpes simplex virus (HSV).
- It is the commonest tumour associated with AIDS.

## Aetiology

- Risk factors include:
  - HSV infection
  - cytomegalovirus infection
  - immunosuppression.

## Pathology

- The tumour is derived from vascular or lymphatic endothelium.

## Clinical features

- Pigmented, non-blanching skin lesions. The lesions are initially red/blue and flat, and later become purple, raised and coalescent. There may be associated bruising and/or lymphoedema.
- Mucocutaneous lesions. Intra-oral lesions account for 15% of clinical presentations.

- Gastrointestinal KS may cause GI bleeding, perforation, intussusception and/or obstruction.
- Pulmonary KS may cause dyspnoea, haemoptysis and/or cough.

# Investigations

- Surgical biopsy.
- HIV testing.
- CD4 count.

# Treatment

- Radiotherapy for lesions on the face, trunk, limbs and penis. The response rate is 60%.
- Intralesional vinblastine is a recognised treatment modality.
- Camouflaging cream.
- Systemic bleomycin, vincristine and steroids for aggressive skin lesions and symptomatic visceral and pulmonary lesions.
- Zidovudine for HIV-infected individuals.
- Surgery for the complications of visceral lesions.

# Prognosis

- This depends on the CD4 count, performance status and the presence of multiple lesions.
- The median survival is 1.5 years from the time of diagnosis.

# 32 Osteosarcoma

## Epidemiology

- This accounts for 3.5% of childhood malignancies.
- It is the commonest primary malignancy of bone.
- The peak incidence occurs in the second decade.
- The male:female ratio is 1.5:1.

## Aetiology

- Ionising radiation.
- Li-Fraumeni syndrome.
- Paget's disease of bone.
- Tumour suppressor genes (e.g. p53) and oncogenes (c-erb B-2, c-fos, MDM2, SAS and CDK4).

## Pathology

- The tumour usually arises in the epiphysis around the knee (lower femur and upper tibia).

## Clinical features

- Pain and swelling around the knee. The swelling is usually tender and warm. There may be limitation of limb movement.
- The plain radiograph usually shows a destructive lesion in the metaphyseal region with new bone formation. There may be elevation of the periosteum (Codman's triangle).

# Investigations

- CT or MRI of the tumour.
- CXR, serum alkaline phosphatase (reflects disease activity), CT of thorax and radioisotope bone scan.

# Management

- This is based on a multi-disciplinary approach involving surgery and chemotherapy.
  - Chemotherapy can be given pre-operatively (neoadjuvant) and/or post-operatively (adjuvant), and has been shown to improve survival.
  - Chemotherapeutic agents used include high-dose methotrexate, cisplatin, doxorubicin, etoposide and ifosfamide.
  - Conservative limb-sparing surgery.
  - Limb-salvage procedures include allograft replacement and endoprosthetic reconstruction.

# Prognosis

- The overall cure rate is 60%.
- Favourable prognostic factors include older age (> 15 years), smaller tumour volume, low histological grade, tibial origin, histological response to chemotherapy and the absence of distant metastases.
- Pulmonary metastases can be resected surgically, with a 3-year survival rate approaching 50%.

# 33 Cutaneous melanoma

## Epidemiology

- The incidence ranges from 0.7 per 100 000 (in black Americans) to 40 per 100 000 (in white Australians) per annum.
- Malignant melanoma accounts for 2.5% of all newly diagnosed cancers.
- The incidence is rising (there has been a 50% rise in the last decade).
- The peak incidence occurs during the fifth decade.

## Aetiology

- Risk factors include:
  - family history of melanoma
  - history of multiple atypical naevi
  - the presence of atypical or numerous naevi
  - inability to tan (fair skin)
  - excessive exposure to ultraviolet radiation
  - immunosuppression
  - genetic factors such as p53 and CDKN2A gene mutations.

## Classification

- Superficial spreading melanoma accounts for 70% of cases.
- Nodular melanoma accounts for 15% of cases.
- Lentigo maligna is uncommon and carries an excellent prognosis.

- Acral lentiginous melanoma represents 10% of all melanomas.
- Amelanotic melanoma. This subtype is difficult to diagnose clinically due to the lack of visual pigmentation. Dermatoscopy may aid the diagnosis.

# Clinical staging system

- **Stage 0: Tis, N0, M0**
  The melanoma is in situ, meaning that it involves the epidermis but has not spread to the dermis (lower layer). This is also called Clark level I.
- **Stage IA: T1a, N0, M0**
  The melanoma is less than 1.0 mm in thickness and Clark level II or III. It is not ulcerated, appears to be localised in the skin, and has not been found in lymph nodes or distant organs.
- **Stage IB: T1b or T2a, N0, M0**
  The melanoma is less than 1.0 mm in thickness and is ulcerated or Clark level IV or V, or it is between 1.01 and 2.0 mm and is not ulcerated. It appears to be localised in the skin and has not been found in lymph nodes or distant organs.
- **Stage IIA: T2b or T3a, N0, M0**
  The melanoma is between 1.01 and 2.0 mm in thickness and is ulcerated, or it is between 2.01 and 4.0 mm and is not ulcerated. It appears to be localised in the skin and has not been found in lymph nodes or distant organs.
- **Stage IIB: T3b or T4a, N0, M0**
  The melanoma is between 2.01 and 4.0 mm in thickness and is ulcerated, or it is thicker than 4.0 mm and is not ulcerated. It appears to be localised in the skin and has not been found in lymph nodes or distant organs.
- **Stage IIC: T4b, N0, M0**
  The melanoma is thicker than 4.0 mm and is ulcerated. It appears to be localised in the skin and has not been found in lymph nodes or distant organs.
- **Stage III: Any T, N1–3, M0**
  The melanoma has spread to lymph nodes near the affected skin area. There is no distant spread. The thickness of the melanoma is

not a factor, although it is usually thick in people with stage III melanoma.

- **Stage IV: Any T, Any N, Any M1**
  The melanoma has spread beyond the original area of skin and nearby lymph nodes to other organs, such as the lung, liver or brain, or to distant areas of the skin or lymph nodes. Neither the lymph node status nor thickness is considered, but in general, the melanoma is thick and has spread to lymph nodes.

# Investigations

- Incisional or excisional biopsy. The latter is preferable if possible.
- FNAC of masses suggestive of metastases (e.g. regional lymph nodes).
- Staging investigations include CXR, liver USS, CT, bone scan and serum lactate dehydrogenase (LDH).

# Treatment

- Primary melanoma is treated by adequate local excision. The defect is closed primarily or using skin grafts and local flaps. The clear margins should be 1 cm for melanoma thickness of < 2 mm and 2–3 cm for melanoma thickness of > 2 mm.
- Lymph nodes.
  - Elective lymph node dissection is performed if the primary melanoma is > 1.5 mm thick and/or there is lymph node involvement.
  - Alternatively, a regional lymph node dissection is performed if the sentinel node is positive for metastatic disease. The sentinel node can be accurately identified (95%) using radioactive isotopes and vital blue dye, and provides an accurate assessment of the regional lymph nodes.
- High-dose interferon-α seems to improve survival in patients with high-risk melanoma.
- Locally advanced/recurrent melanoma is treated by hyperthermic isolated limb perfusion (e.g. with melphalan), with a remission rate of 40%.

- Distant metastases.
  - Systemic chemotherapy using dacarbazine (20–25% response rate).
  - Solitary or limited numbers of metastases in the brain, intestine or lungs can be resected with prolongation of survival.
  - Immunotherapy (e.g. with interferon-$\alpha$) has a 15–20% response rate. Vaccination, anti-tumour vaccines, monoclonal antibodies and high-dose interleukin-2 (IL-2) are still under investigation.
  - Radiotherapy for palliation of inoperable brain, lymph node and bone metastases.

# Follow-up

- Stage IA patients should be reviewed 6-monthly for 2 years, and then yearly.
- Stage IB and IIA patients should be reviewed 4-monthly for 3 years, and then yearly.
- Stage IIB and III patients should be reviewed 4-monthly for 5 years, and then yearly.
- Patients should be educated in self-examination.

# Prognosis

- This depends upon tumour stage, thickness and the presence of ulceration, the patient's age and sex, the primary lesion site and the growth pattern.
- The 5-year survival rate is 90–95% for stage I; 85% for stage IIA; 73% for stage IIB; 53% for stage IIC; 45% for stage III; 10% for stage IV.

# 34 Non-melanocytic skin cancer

## Epidemiology

- This is the commonest cancer among Caucasians in the UK and the USA.
- Its incidence is increasing.
- The incidence is slightly higher in men (especially above the age of 70 years).

## Aetiology

- Actinic radiation.
- Chronic skin ulcers and sinuses.
- Immunosuppression.
- Genetic predisposition, including xeroderma pigmentosum, multiple familial self-healing squamous-cell carcinoma and Gorlin–Goltz syndrome (basal-cell carcinoma).
- Bowen's disease predisposes to squamous-cell carcinoma.

## Pathology

- Basal-cell carcinoma (BCC) usually invades locally. Regional lymph node involvement is extremely rare.
- Squamous-cell carcinoma (SCC) systemic spread occurs in 2% of cases.

# Clinical features

- A skin ulcer. The ulcer margins may be rolled (in SCC) or pearly and everted (in BCC). Surface telangiectasia may be present (in BCC).
- A skin nodule or cystic lesion.
- The skin lesion is occasionally pigmented.
- Regional lymphadenopathy (in SCC).

# Investigations

- Excisional biopsy.
- Incisional biopsy.
- Shaving biopsy.
- FNAC of enlarged lymph nodes.

# Treatment

- Adequate surgical excision with a minimal margin of 4 mm for BCC and 1 cm for SCC. The surgical defect can be closed primarily or using a skin graft, a local flap or a myocutaneous flap (conventional or free transfer).
- Radiotherapy is an effective treatment modality.
- Regional lymph node dissection or radiotherapy is used for involved nodes.
- Other treatment modalities include cryosurgery, laser therapy, curettage or electro-desiccation.

# Prognosis

- The 5-year survival rate is 98% for SCC and 100% for BCC.
- Death from BCC is extremely rare.
- The 5-year incidence of further BCC lesions is 40%.

# 35 Ovarian cancer

## Epidemiology

- This accounts for 25% of all gynaecological malignancies.
- The incidence is 22.8 per 100 000 per annum in the UK.
- The peak incidence occurs in the age range 40–60 years.

## Aetiology

- Risk factors include:
  - late menopause
  - family history of ovarian, endometrial, breast or bowel cancer
  - nulliparity
  - late first pregnancy
  - use of peritoneal talc
  - BRCA-1 gene.

## Pathology

- Epithelial carcinoma accounts for 90% of cases.
- Exfoliation through the peritoneal cavity and lymphatic spread are the commonest modes of dissemination.

## Clinical features

- Irregular periods.
- Abnormal vaginal bleeding.
- Abdominal pain (50% of cases).

- Urinary or bowel symptoms.
- Ascites.
- Abdominal distension.
- Dyspareunia and anorexia.
- Pelvic mass.
- Constitutional symptoms (50% of cases).

# Investigations

- Abdomino-pelvic US, CT or MRI scan.
- Serum CA125, α-fetoprotein (AFP) and human chorionic gonadotrophin (HCG).
- CXR, IVU and barium enema.
- Laparoscopy.
- Laparotomy/biopsies.

# Treatment

- Early-stage disease confined to the ovary can be treated by total abdominal hysterectomy and bilateral salpingo-oophorectomy (BSO), infracolic omentectomy and surgical staging. Systemic chemotherapy is required for poorly-differentiated (grade 3) tumours.
- Advanced-stage disease is treated by debulking surgery that aims to reduce the disease to < 1.5 cm tumour followed by chemotherapy (cisplatinum and paclitaxel for 6 cycles).
- Recurrent disease is treated by chemotherapy (e.g. with liposomal doxorubicin or topotecan) and/or radiotherapy.
- Germ-cell tumours in the young are treated by chemotherapy following surgical staging.

# Prognosis

- The 5-year survival rate is 88% for stage I lesions (lesions confined to the ovary), 70% for stage II lesions (lesions extending to the pelvis only) and 20% for advanced disease.

# Future directions

- The role of angiogenesis inhibitors (angiostatin, endostatin, thalidomide and EGFR antagonists), COX-2 inhibitors, Herceptin in patients with HER2-positive tumours (10%), photodynamic therapy and immune modulation is currently being evaluated in patients with advanced and recurrent disease.
- Serum proteomics using mass spectrometry seems to be promising in the early detection of ovarian cancer.

# 36 Endometrial carcinoma

## Epidemiology

- Endometrial carcinoma is one of the commonest gynaecological malignancy.
- Its incidence has been increasing.
- The median age of onset is 60 years.
- Around 20% of cases occur before the menopause.
- The incidence is low in Nigeria (0.6 per 100 000 women) and high in the UK (18.7 per 100 000 women).

## Aetiology

- Risk factors include:
  - obesity
  - late menopause
  - diabetes mellitus
  - nulliparity
  - unopposed oestrogen exposure
  - tamoxifen therapy.

## Pathology

- Adenocarcinoma is the commonest type (90% of cases).
- Other histopathological types include adenoacanthoma, adenosquamous and leiomyosarcoma.
- Direct extension is the commonest mode of spread.

# Clinical features

- Abnormal vaginal bleeding (90% of cases).
- Abnormal cervical smear cytology.
- Symptoms and signs of metastases.

# Investigations

- Cervical smear cytology and endocervical curettage.
- Endometrial biopsy.
- Dilatation and curettage.
- Hysteroscopy.
- Staging investigations include FBC, LFTs, U&Es, CXR, IVP, abdomino-pelvic CT or MRI and/or bone scan (if indicated).

# Staging (FIGO)

- Stage I:
  - IA – tumour limited to the endometrium
  - IB – invasion of < 50% of myometrium
  - IC – invasion of > 50% of myometrium.
- Stage II:
  - IIA – endocervical glandular involvement only
  - IIB – cervical stromal invasion.
- Stage III:
  - IIIA – tumour invades serosa/positive peritoneal washings
  - IIIB – vaginal metastases
  - IIIC – metastases to pelvic/aortic lymph nodes.
- Stage IV:
  - IVA – invasion of bowel/bladder mucosa
  - IVB – distant metastases.

# Treatment

- Stage I and II disease is treated by total abdominal hysterectomy and bilateral salpingo-oophorectomy (BSO). Pelvic and para-aortic lymph nodes are sampled. Radiotherapy is indicated for poorly differentiated carcinoma (grade III).
- Stage IC, IIA and IIB lesions. Large stage I lesions may be treated by pre-operative radiotherapy followed by hysterectomy and BSO 6 weeks later.
- Advanced and recurrent lesions are treated by a combination of surgery, radiotherapy, chemotherapy (doxorubicin) and hormonal manipulation.
- Hormonal manipulation includes megestrol acetate (80 mg twice a day), medroxyprogesterone acetate (50 mg three times a day) and anti-oestrogens.

# Prognosis

- The 5-year survival rate is 73% for stage I, 56% for stage II, 30% for stage III and 10% for stage IV.

# 37 Cervical cancer

## Epidemiology

- Cervical cancer is the second cause of female malignancy worldwide.
- A total of 13 500 new cases are diagnosed in the USA every year.
- The average age of onset is 45 years.
- The incidence is declining.

## Aetiology

- Risk factors include cervical intra-epithelial neoplasia (CIN), young age at first intercourse, high parity, low socio-economic status, human papilloma virus (HPV) infection (types 16, 18, 31, 33 and 35), smoking, venereal infections and multiple sexual partners.

## Pathology

- Squamous-cell carcinoma (SCC) accounts for 80% of cases.
- Adenocarcinoma and adenosquamous lesions account for 20% of cases.

## Clinical features

- Vaginal discharge.

- Abnormal vaginal bleeding (post-coital, post-menopausal or irregular) is present in 85% of cases.
- Abnormal routine cervical smear.
- The cervical tumour may be ulcerative, necrotic, exophytic or granular in appearance.
- Pelvic mass.
- Ureteric obstruction in advanced disease.
- Signs and symptoms of metastases (e.g. ascites and inguinal lymphadenopathy).

# Investigations

- Cervical cytology (Pap smear).
- Colposcopy plus biopsy or endocervical curettage or conisation.
- Cystoscopy and IVP.
- Sigmoidoscopy/barium enema.
- CXR (lung metastases are present in 5% of cases).
- Abdomino-pelvic CT or MRI scan.
- Bone scan.
- Combined vaginal and rectal examination under anaesthesia.
- FBC, serum U&Es and LFTs.

# Staging (FIGO)

- Stage 0:  carcinoma *in situ.*
- Stage I:  carcinoma is confined to the cervix.
- Stage II: carcinoma extends beyond the cervix, but has not extended to the pelvic wall or the lower third of the vagina.
- Stage III: carcinoma has extended to the pelvic wall or the lower third of the vagina.
- Stage IVA: carcinoma has extended beyond the pelvic wall or has involved the rectal/vesical mucosa clinically.
- Stage IVB: carcinoma is palliated by radiotherapy and chemotherapy.

# Treatment

- CIN is managed by colposcopy and cryosurgery, $CO_2$ laser, electrocoagulation, loop electrodiathermy or cervical conisation. CIN stage II may be cured by hysterectomy in patients who have completed childbearing.
- Microinvasive disease (stage IA) can be treated by a cone biopsy (with clear margins) or extrafascial abdominal hysterectomy.
- Stage IB and IIA tumours are treated by radical hysterectomy with excision of parametrial tissue, vaginal cuff, lymphadenectomy and sampling of the para-aortic nodes and/or radiotherapy (external beam followed by intracavity radiation). Surgery is superior to radiotherapy for adenocarcinoma.
- Stage IB, IIA and IIB lesions are treated by radiotherapy (external beam followed by intracavity radiotherapy).
- Stage IVA carcinoma is treated by pelvic radiotherapy. Salvage pelvic extenteration is reserved for partially responding tumours.
- Recurrent disease is treated by chemotherapy (mitomycin C, methotrexate, cyclophosphamide, bleomycin and cis-platinum), pelvic extenteration and/or radiotherapy.

# Prognosis

- The 5-year survival rate is 75% for stage I, 55% for stage II, 30% for stage III and 7% for stage IV lesions.

# Screening

- All women, once they have become sexually active, should undergo an annual physical examination and Papanicolaou smear of the cervix.
- The false-negative rate for cervical cytology is 15% and the false-positive rate is less than 1%.

# Future prospects

- Serum proteomics using mass spectrometry seems to be promising in the early detection of cervical cancer.
- Cervical cancer vaccines based on HPV are likely to be available for clinical use within the next 5 years.

# 38 Vaginal cancer

## Epidemiology

- Primary vaginal cancer accounts for 1.5% of all gynaecological malignancies.
- The highest incidence occurs in the age range 50–70 years.
- Most lesions occur in the upper third of the vagina.

## Aetiology

- Maternal ingestion of diethylstilboestrol during pregnancy increases the incidence of vaginal clear-cell carcinoma in daughters.
- Vaginal intra-epithelial neoplasia has a pre-malignant potential.
- Other risk factors include:
  - vaginal pessaries
  - venereal disease
  - human papilloma virus (HPV) infection
  - procidentia
  - ulceration
  - cervical cancer.

## Pathology

- Squamous-cell carcinoma (SCC) accounts for 93% of cases and adenocarcinoma accounts for 5% of cases.
- Embryonal rhabdomyosarcomas are seen in children.

# Clinical features

- Vaginal bleeding/discharge.
- Ulcerative/exophytic vaginal lesions.
- Urinary and gastrointestinal symptoms are occasionally seen.
- Regional lymphadenopathy (inguinal, femoral and obturator).
- Abnormal cervical smear.

# Investigations

- Punch biopsy.
- Colposcopy and endometrial curettage.
- CXR.
- Cystoscopy and IVP.
- Abdomino-pelvic CT or MRI scanning.
- Sigmoidoscopy and/or barium enema.
- FNAC of enlarged lymph nodes.

# Staging (FIGO)

- Stage I: tumour confined to the vaginal wall.
- Stage II: tumour has involved subvaginal tissue but has not extended to the pelvic wall.
- Stage III: tumour has extended to the pelvic wall.
- Stage IV: tumour has extended beyond the pelvic wall or has involved the rectal or vesicle mucosa.

# Treatment

- Radiotherapy (external beam radiation or interstitial) is the mainstay of management. The groins are included in the radiotherapy field for tumours arising in the lower third of the vagina.

- Surgery in the form of a wide local excision or total vaginectomy is indicated for early vaginal cancer. Radical surgery may entail hysterectomy and pelvic lymphadenopathy.
- Psychological counselling is essential prior to vaginectomy.
- A neovagina may be reconstructed using a split-thickness skin graft.
- Surgery is indicated for recurrent tumours following radiotherapy.

# Prognosis

- The 5-year survival rate is 87% for stage I, 60% for stage II, 33% for stage III and 7% for stage IV tumours.
- Around 10% of patients develop significant bowel and bladder side-effects following radiotherapy.

# 39 Vulval cancer

## Epidemiology

- Vulval cancer accounts for 4% of all gynaecological cancers.
- The incidence is highest during the seventh decade of life.

## Aetiology

- Risk factors include immunosuppression, vulval dystrophy and human papilloma virus infection.

## Pathology

- Squamous-cell carcinoma accounts for 85% of cases.
- Melanoma accounts for 5% of cases.

## Clinical features

- Vulval pruritus/pain.
- Vulval ulcer/mass.
- Inguinal lymphadenopathy.

## Investigations

- Surgical biopsy.
- FNAC of regional lymph nodes (if enlarged).
- Abdomino-pelvic CT or MRI for staging.

# Treatment

- Carcinoma *in situ* and microinvasive disease are managed by local vulval excision with a clear margin of 1 cm.
- Lateral cancers less than 2 cm in diameter are managed by vulvectomy (with a 2 cm clear margin) and ipsilateral lymph node dissection. A contralateral lymph node dissection is recommended if the ipsilateral nodes are involved.
- Bilateral inguinal lymph node dissection is indicated for vulval cancer involving the clitoris.
- Pelvic lymphadenectomy is recommended for lesions over 4 cm in diameter.
- The terminal urethra can be excised in order to achieve adequate local excision.
- Butterfly or triple incision is used for vulvectomy and inguinal node dissection. Skin flaps are created to relieve tension. Deep vein thrombosis (DVT) and antimicrobial prophylaxis is essential.
- Compression stockings and lymphoedema play an important role after inguinal node dissection (the incidence of lymphoedema is 60%).
- Radiotherapy can be given pre-operatively to render large lesions operable. Other indications include inadequate margins and recurrent disease.
- Chemotherapy (bleomycin and methotrexate) has a minor role.

# 40 Renal adenocarcinoma

## Epidemiology

- This accounts for 3% of all adult cancers.
- The male:female ratio is 2:1.
- The peak incidence occurs in the age range 40–60 years.

## Aetiology

- Risk factors include Hippel–Lindau syndrome, smoking, exposure to cadmium, and polycystic kidneys of patients on renal dialysis.

## Pathology

- Polygonal or round cells with abundant cytoplasm are characteristic.
- Haematogenous spread is the principal mode of metastasis.

## Clinical features

- The main symptoms are loin pain (40% of cases), haematuria (40%), abdominal mass (25%) and weight loss (35%).
- Other features include varicocoele, hypercalcaemia, polycythaemia, hypertension and night sweating.

# Investigations

- Urine microscopy and culture, FBC, serum, U&Es, serum calcium and CXR.
- IVU.
- Ultrasonography.
- CT or MRI scanning.
- Bone scan.

# Treatment

- Total nephrectomy with perinephric fat and Gerota's fascia after early control and division of renal vessels through an anterior approach. Lymph node dissection has a low yield of metastasis (3%).
- Partial nephrectomy for small cortical tumours and bilateral lesions.
- Palliation of metastatic disease includes analgesia, Provera (100 mg three times a day), radiotherapy to bone secondaries and radiological embolisation for intractable haematuria.
- Interferon-α is indicated for selected patients with metastatic disease (response rate is around 15%). It prolongs life by 5 months.
- The role of interleukin-2 (IL-2), gene therapy and immuno-therapy is currently under investigation.

# Prognosis

- The 5-year survival rate is 70% if the tumour is confined within the capsule, 45% if the tumour has breached Gerota's fascia and 30% if there is regional lymph node involvement.

# 41 Wilms' tumour

## Epidemiology

- This accounts for 6% of all childhood malignancies.
- The peak incidence occurs between 3 and 4 years of age.

## Pathology

- It may be multifocal and bilateral (5%).
- Mesodermal, mesonephric and metanephric origins have been proposed for this tumour.

## Clinical features

- Abdominal mass, anorexia, haematuria and/or hypertension.
- Associated congenital abnormalities include aniridia, hemi-hypertrophy, cryptorchidism and Beckwith's syndrome.

## Investigations

- Abdominal USS or CT.
- CXR.
- Renogram.
- Doppler examination of the renal vein and inferior vena cava.

# Staging

- Stage I: tumour is confined to the kidney and completely excised.
- Stage II: tumour extends beyond the renal capsule but is completely excised.
- Stage III: tumour is inoperable, incompletely excised or ruptured diffusely during removal.
- Stage IV: distant metastases are present.
- Stage V: tumour is bilateral.

# Treatment

- Surgical debulking of the tumour should be undertaken if possible (nephrectomy).
- Radiotherapy and chemotherapy (vincristine and actinomycin D for stages I and II; vincristine, actinomycin and adriamycin for stages III, IV and V).
- Chemotherapy is given pre-operatively in stages IV and V.
- Radiotherapy is indicated in stages III, IV and V.

# Prognosis

- The 5-year survival rate is 95% for stages I and II, 82% for stage III, 60% for stage IV and 67% for stage V.

# 42 Urothelial carcinoma

## Epidemiology

- The incidence is 17 per 100 000 per annum.
- The male:female ratio is 3:1.
- It is more common in industrialised countries.

## Aetiology

- Risk factors include smoking and occupational hazards (rubber, aniline dye and plastics industries, tyre destruction and cable production).
- Genetic abnormalities and oncogenes (ras and C-myc) have been implicated.
- Balkan nephropathy.
- Drugs (e.g. phenacetin and cyclophosphamide).

## Pathology

- Around 95% of lesions affect the bladder.
- Transitional-cell carcinomas (TCC) can be subdivided into carcinoma *in situ* (CIS), superficial and deep disease (involving muscle).

# Clinical features

- Haematuria is the commonest symptom.
- Other symptoms include loin pain, urinary tract infection, weight loss, back pain and jaundice.
- Signs include renal and pelvic masses.

# Investigations

- Urine microscopy and culture.
- Urine cytology and proteomics (NMP22).
- IVU and flexible cystoscopy.
- Diagnostic cystoscopy (under general anaesthetic) and biopsy.
- USS, CT or MRI.
- Other investigations include LFTs, bone scan, CXR and laparoscopic sampling of pelvic lymph nodes.

# Treatment and prognosis

- TCC of the renal pelvis and ureter is treated by radical nephro-ureterectomy if the tumour is poorly differentiated or has invaded muscle. Segmental resection and end-to-end anastomosis is suitable for well-differentiated and superficial tumours. Urethroscopic laser therapy may be used to treat small tumours. The median survival is 1 year for invasive tumours and 7 years for non-invasive tumours.
- Superficial TCC is treated by endoscopic transurethral resection and surveillance.
- Intravesical chemotherapy (mitomycin and epirubicin) and immunotherapy (BCG, bacille Calmette–Guérin) are suitable for frequent and numerous recurrences.
- Radical cystectomy is considered for high-grade tumours with lamina propria invasion, particularly if there is coexistent CIS.
- Primary CIS of the bladder is treated with intravesical mitomycin and BCG in order to prevent aggressive disease. Recurrence or failure to respond to the above treatment is an indication for cystectomy.

- Invasive TCC of the bladder.
  - Patients with localised disease are offered radical cystectomy. The 5-year survival rate is 40%.
  - A catheterisable or continent neobladder (e.g. hemi-Koch pouch) is usually constructed after radical cystectomy.
  - Radical cystectomy entails the removal of the regional lymph nodes and prostate or uterus and anterior vaginal wall.
  - Patients with metastases are treated palliatively. Palliation includes radiotherapy, chemotherapy and/or cystectomy. The 2-year survival rate is 5%.

# 43 Prostatic adenocarcinoma

## Epidemiology

- The incidence is 75 per 100 000 per annum and is rising due to ageing populations.
- Men have a 10% lifetime risk of developing the disease and a 3% risk of dying from it.
- The incidence is relatively high among American Negroes and is low in Japan.

## Aetiology

- Genetic and environmental factors (e.g. selenium deficiency) have been implicated.

## Pathology

- Most carcinomas arise in the peripheral zone.
- Haematogenous spread occurs predominantly to bone (sclerotic lesions) and lymphatic spread occurs to pelvic nodes.

## Clinical features

- Bladder outflow obstruction (urgency, frequency, nocturia, urinary retention and hesitancy).
- Incidental findings in TURP specimens.

- Mass detected on digital rectal examination.
- Bony pain due to metastases.
- Haematuria.

# Investigations

- Serum prostate-specific antigen (PSA) (normal range is < 4 ng/ml). PSA is elevated in prostatic cancer, benign prostatic hyperplasia, prostatitis and urinary retention. It is useful for indicating recurrence (after prostatectomy) and bony metastases.
- Transrectal ultrasonography and biopsy.
- Bone scan and pelvic CT and/or MRI may be indicated.

# Treatment and prognosis

- Total prostatectomy.
  - This is indicated for tumours that are confined to the prostate.
  - The procedure cures all impalpable lesions confined to the prostate (T1) and 35% of palpable tumours which appear to be confined to the prostate (T2).
  - The incidence of incontinence should be less than 5% and that of impotence less than 20%. The incidence of impotence is higher if a nerve-sparing technique is not adopted.
  - The procedure can be performed laparoscopically with three-dimensional viewing and magnification. This approach seems to be associated with shorter hospitalisation times and lower morbidity rates.
- Radiotherapy (external beam or interstitial).
  - This is indicated for tumours that are confined to the prostate (T1 and T2). The 5-year survival rate is approximately 65–70%.
  - Radiotherapy achieves similar survival rates to surgery.
  - It is also used to palliate bony pain due to metastases and prostatic bleeding.
- Hormonal manipulation.
  - This is indicated for metastatic disease. Around 80% of tumours are sensitive to androgen deprivation.

  – Modalities available include diethylstilboestrol (1 mg daily), bicalutamide, cyproterone acetate, flutamide, luteinising hormone-releasing hormone analogues (e.g. goserelin) and orchidectomy (subcapsular or total). These modalities can be used singly or in combination.
  – The median survival for metastatic disease is 30 months.
● Bone metastases.
  – Hormonal manipulation.
  – External beam radiation.
  – Strontium-89 chloride (systemic radionuclide therapy).
  – Bisphosphonates.

# Future prospects

● Serum proteomics using mass spectrometry seems to be promising in the early detection of prostate cancer. Early results suggest that this test is more accurate than serum PSA.
● Computer-assisted endoscopic surgery is likely to become the standard surgical treatment for early prostate cancer.

# 44 Testicular cancer

## Epidemiology

- The incidence is rising (e.g. 8 per 100 000 per year in Denmark).
- The peak incidence occurs between 20 and 34 years of age.
- The lifetime risk in Caucasians is 0.2%.
- The incidence is lower among Asians.

## Aetiology

- Risk factors include:
  - cryptorchidism
  - oestrogen exposure
  - testicular torsion
  - mumps
  - orchitis
  - testicular trauma, including open biopsy
  - infertility
  - early puberty
  - lack of exercise
  - orchidectomy
  - low sperm counts
  - elevated levels of follicle-stimulating hormone (FSH).
- It is likely that the FSH-driven over-stimulation of spermatogonia is the underlying mechanism for some of the above factors.

# Pathology

- Testicular germ-cell tumours account for 95% of cases.
- Histological subclasses include spermatocytic seminoma (classical and anaplastic), teratoma (differentiated, intermediate and undifferentiated), embryonal carcinoma, choriocarcinoma (pure and mixed) and yolk-sac tumour.
- Carcinoma *in situ* (CIS) is a universal precursor.

# Clinical features

- Scrotal mass (painless in 75% of cases).
- Solid mass that cannot be distinguished from the testis.
- Secondary hydrocoele.
- Lymphadenopathy (abdominal or cervical).
- Gynaecomastia.
- Symptoms due to metastases (e.g. backache).

# Investigations

- Ultrasonography.
- Serum tumour markers ($\alpha$-fetoprotein, human chorionic gonadotrophin and lactate dehydrogenase). These remain important for diagnosis, and they have prognostic value and can be used to monitor therapy and follow-up.
- Orchidectomy (via inguinal approach) for histological examination.
- Staging investigations including CXR, CT (thorax and abdomen), lymphangiography, abdominal ultrasound and/or FNAC of extra-scrotal masses. The false-negative rate for CT staging is 25%.
- PET scanning is useful for staging the disease in selected patients.

# Treatment and prognosis

- Stage I seminoma is treated by total orchidectomy plus adjuvant chemotherapy (one or two courses of carboplatin) or radiotherapy. The disease-free survival rate is 98–100%. Some centres recommend long-term surveillance only and omit adjuvant therapy.
- For stage I seminoma, adjuvant carboplatin chemotherapy offers a similar disease-free survival rate to adjuvant radiotherapy.
- Stage I non-seminoma is treated by total orchidectomy plus nerve-sparing retroperitoneal lymph node dissection (RPLND). Adjuvant chemotherapy is given to patients with poor histological indicators (e.g. vascular invasion and anaplastic changes). The survival rate is 98% and the relapse rate is 5%.
- Stage II seminoma is treated by radiotherapy or chemotherapy (with carboplatin or etoposide/platinum).
- Stage II non-seminoma is treated by orchidectomy, RPLND and chemotherapy (with bleomycin/etoposide/platinum).
- Stage III/IV seminoma and non-seminoma are treated primarily with multiple courses of chemotherapy (bleomycin/etoposide/cisplatin). Surgical excision of metastases is performed in any patient with residual disease after tumour markers have been negative for more than 6 weeks. The primary cure rate is 85%.
- Brain metastases of testicular germ-cell tumours are treated with a combination of chemotherapy and cranial irradiation.

# 45 Squamous-cell carcinoma of the penis

## Epidemiology

- This accounts for less than 1% of all male cancers in the developed world.
- It is rare in males who have been circumcised at birth or during childhood.

## Aetiology

- Circumcision prevents squamous-cell carcinoma (SCC) of the penis.
- Pre-malignant lesions include Paget's disease, De Queryrat's erythroplasia and Bowen's disease of the glans penis.

## Pathology

- Stage I: tumour is confined to the glans or prepuce.
- Stage II: tumour involves the penile shaft.
- Stage III: there is regional node involvement.
- Stage IV: the nodes are fixed.

# Clinical features

- An ulcer or reddened area on the glans.
- Purulent discharge.
- Inguinal lymphadenopathy.

# Investigations

- Surgical biopsy.
- FNAC of enlarged inguinal nodes.
- Pelvic CT for staging.

# Treatment

- Stage I is treated with radiotherapy (external beam or interstitial). If this fails, partial penile amputation is performed. Superficial lesions can be ablated by laser therapy.
- Stage II is treated with partial or total penile amputation. Perineal urethrostomy may be performed.
- Stage III is treated with radical phallectomy and regional lymphadenopathy (one testis should be preserved).
- Stage IV may be palliated with toilet surgery.
- The sentinel-node biopsy can be performed in order to stage the disease.

# Prognosis

- The 5-year survival rate is 80% for well-differentiated tumours and 20% for poorly differentiated ones.

# 46 Primary intracranial tumours

## Epidemiology

- The incidence is 4 per 100 000 of the general population per year.
- They are the second commonest malignancy in children (after leukaemia).
- There are two peaks of incidence (in the first decade and in the fifth/sixth decades).

## Aetiology

- Genetic factors. CNS tumours are a major component of some inherited conditions such as tuberous sclerosis, neurofibromatosis and von Hippel–Lindau syndrome.
- Radiation.
- Immunosuppression.

## Pathology

- CNS tumours can be classified according to cell origin as glioma (the commonest type), medulloblastoma, neuroblastoma, meningioma, schwannoma, neurofibroma and lymphoma.
- Gliomas include astrocytoma, oligodendroglioma, ependymoma and glioblastoma multiforme.

# Clinical features

- Symptoms and signs due to the local effects of the tumour on the surrounding structures, which are destroyed or impaired due to infiltration, mechanical pressure and/or oedema.
- Symptoms and signs of raised intracranial pressure (e.g. headaches, vomiting and papilloedema).
- Shifting of the intracranial contents can cause compression of the brainstem and false localising signs.
- Seizures (complex, partial or simple).
- Progressive deterioration is the hallmark of clinical presentation.

# Investigations

- MRI or CT scan.
- Skull X-rays are useful in pituitary and parasellar regions.
- Technetium brain scan may confirm the site of the lesion.
- Stereotactic or CT-guided biopsy.
- Other tests include an EEG, angiography and ventriculography.

# Treatment and prognosis

- Low-grade astrocytomas are treated by surgical excision followed by radiotherapy (external beam, interstitial or stereotactic) and chemotherapy (with carmustine, lomustine, procarbazine, cisplatin and vincristine).
- Ependymoma is treated with radiotherapy to the primary tumour site (50 Gy over a period of 4–5 weeks). Craniospinal radiation is indicated for high-grade tumours. The overall 5-year survival rate is 40%.
- Oligodendroglioma is treated with surgical excision and postoperative radiotherapy. Chemotherapy is indicated for recurrent disease. The 10-year survival rate is 35%.
- Deep-seated gliomas are treated with radiotherapy (50 Gy over a period of 4–5 weeks).

- Medulloblastoma is treated with surgical excision (if possible) and radiotherapy. The latter consists of brain irradiation down to the level of C2 (30 Gy over a period of 3 weeks), a boosting dose to the posterior cranial fossa and mid-brain and spinal irradiation. Chemotherapy is indicated in young children and in patients with recurrent disease.
- Meningioma is treated by complete surgical excision. If this is not possible due to its location, radiotherapy (55 Gy over a period of 5–6 weeks) is used. This tumour is curable.
- Pituitary tumours are treated by trans-sphenoidal excision (if there is no suprasellar extension) or excision through a craniotomy (if the tumour extends outside the pituitary fossa). Post-operative radiotherapy can be given. Prolactinomas may be treated with bromocriptine.
- Acoustic neuroma is treated by surgical excision.
- Seizures are treated with anticonvulsants (e.g. phenytoin).
- Cerebral oedema may be treated with corticosteroids (e.g. dexamethasone) and osmotic diuretics (e.g. mannitol or urea).
- Hydrocephalus can be treated with surgical decompression using ventriculo-peritoneal or ventriculo-atrial shunts.

# 47 Cerebral metastases

## Epidemiology

- Around 30% of patients with systemic cancer have cerebral metastases.
- The metastases are solitary in 50% of cases and multiple in the remaining 50% of cases.

## Pathology

- The common primaries include breast, bronchus, melanoma, lymphoma and prostate.
- Spread is usually haematogenous.
- The metastasis is usually surrounded by cerebral oedema.
- Haemorrhage may occur within metastases (e.g. in melanoma).

## Clinical features

- Epilepsy, focal neurological deficit, raised intracranial pressure (ICP) and cerebellar symptoms and signs.

## Investigations

- MRI is the investigation of choice.
- Contrast-enhanced CT.
- Needle biopsy (under stereotactic guidance).
- Investigations of the primary lesion.

# Treatment

- Surgical excision is indicated for surgically accessible solitary metastases in the absence of apparent systemic disease in fit patients. Dexamethasone (4 mg four times a day for 2 days) and post-operative radiotherapy are given. The median survival is 2 years.
- Whole-brain radiotherapy (35 Gy) and/or steroids are indicated for multiple metastases or surgically inaccessible lesions.

# Prognosis

- The overall median survival is 6 months.

# 48 Spinal metastases

## Epidemiology

- Spinal metastases are found in 30% of patients dying of cancer.
- The thoracic spine is the commonest site.

## Pathology

- The common primaries include breast, bronchus, kidney, thyroid, prostate and haematological malignancies.
- Modes of spread include haematogenous spread (the commonest), direct extension, perineural and lymphatic spread.
- Metastases may cause bony destruction, cord compression and deformity, spinal oedema, ischaemia and/or infarction.
- The metastases may be extradural (the commonest type), intradural/extramedullary or intradural/intramedullary.

## Clinical features

- Pain (spinal or radicular).
- Urinary retention.
- Spastic paraplegia.
- Brown–Sequard's syndrome.
- Neurological symptoms and signs depending upon the degree of spinal involvement.

# Investigations

- FBC, erythrocyte sedimentation rate (ESR), LFTs, serum electrophoresis and serum biochemistry.
- CXR and plain radiographs of the spine.
- MRI is the investigation of choice.
- Myelography.
- CT (with or without myelography).
- CT-guided biopsy if the primary is unknown.
- Investigations for the primary lesion.

# Treatment

- High-dose steroids to reduce the symptoms of cord compression and oedema.
- Radiotherapy is effective in relieving cord compression and pain.
- Anterior spinal decompression or laminectomy is considered if there is neurological deterioration despite the radiotherapy, and in relatively fit patients with a good prognosis. Complete paraplegia lasting more than 24 hours is a contraindication.
- The vertebral body can be reconstructed following anterior decompression using methyl methacrylate and Steinmann's pins or iliac bone grafts.
- Posterior stabilisation of the spine may be performed following decompression.
- Anterior decompression can be performed through a thoracotomy, thoraco-abdominal retroperitoneal or transperitoneal approach, depending upon the site of compression.

# Primary spinal cord tumours

- Primary tumours of the spinal cord are uncommon.
- Ependymoma is the commonest tumour. Meningiomas and schwannomas are relatively common, whereas astrocytomas are rare.

- Treatment consists of high-dose dexamethasone, surgical excision of the tumour (if possible) and post-operative radiotherapy. Spinal cord decompression should be performed (when indicated) even if the tumour is thought to be unresectable.

# 49 Acute leukaemia

## Epidemiology

- The incidence of acute myeloid leukaemia (AML) rises with age (to 15 per 100 000 during the eighth decade).
- Acute lymphoblastic leukaemia (ALL) accounts for 80% of leukaemias during childhood (3 per 100 000 during the first decade).
- AML accounts for 85% of leukaemias after the second decade.
- The male:female ratio is 3:2.

## Aetiology

- Ionising radiation.
- Benzene exposure.
- Cytotoxic chemotherapy.
- Occupational exposure (e.g. welding, DDT industries).
- Smoking increases the risk by 50%.
- Inherited syndromes (e.g. Down's syndrome, Bloom's syndrome, Fanconi's anaemia, ataxia telangiectasia).
- Specific chromosomal abnormalities (e.g. t(8;21), t(15;17), t(9;11), t(4;11), etc.).
- Oncogene expression (e.g. N-ras and WT1 in AML).
- Viruses.

# Pathology and classification

## Morphological classification of acute leukaemia

- ALL:
  - $L_1$: small monomorphic cells (scanty cytoplasm and fewer nucleoli)
  - $L_2$: large heterogeneous cells (more common in adults)
  - $L_3$: Burkitt type.
- AML:
  - $M_1$: myeloblastic (no maturation)
  - $M_2$: myeloblastic (some maturation)
  - $M_3$: promyelocytic
  - $M_4$: myelomonocytic
  - $M_5$: monocytic
  - $M_6$: erythroleukaemia
  - $M_7$: megakaryoblastic.
- Cytochemical staining helps to determine the type of leukaemia in doubtful cases.
- Immunological classification of leukaemia assists understanding of the pathogenesis of the disease.

# Clinical features

- ALL.
  - The symptoms include malaise, fever, bone pains, oral and pharyngeal ulceration and petechiae.
  - The signs include pallor, lymphadenopathy, hepatosplenomegaly, haemorrhages and bone tenderness. Mediastinal masses are more common in adults.
  - Symptoms and signs of malignant meningitis are occasionally present.
- AML.
  - The clinical features are similar to those of ALL.

- Bone pain, lymphadenopathy and CNS involvement are less common than in ALL.
- Gum hypertrophy is relatively common in $M_4$ and $M_5$.

# Investigations

- FBC may reveal anaemia, thrombocytopenia and leukocytosis. Lymphoblasts or myeloblasts are usually present. The white blood count (WBC) may not be elevated.
- Bone-marrow examination must show more than 30% blast cells.
- Cytochemical staining and immunological typing are used when appropriate.
- Serum biochemistry.
- Clotting screen.
- CXR may show a mediastinal mass, especially in T-cell leukaemia, due to thymic enlargement.
- Plain radiographs may show osteolytic lesions, demineralisation and/or radiolucent bands in the metaphysis.
- Lumbar puncture should be performed if indicated.

# Treatment

- ALL.
  - Remission induction is achieved by means of vincristine, prednisolone and doxorubicin, followed by an intensive consolidation regimen consisting of doxorubicin, asparaginase, methotrexate and cytosine arabinoside.
  - CNS prophylaxis consists of cranial radiation (18 Gy in 10 fractions over 2 weeks) plus intrathecal methotrexate. CNS disease is treated by craniospinal radiation (24 Gy over 2 weeks).
  - Testicular disease is treated by radiotherapy (24 Gy over 2 weeks).
  - Maintenance therapy is continued for 2 years. Methotrexate, vincristine, prednisolone and mercaptopurine are used.

- Relapse within the first year of treatment is an indication for bone-marrow transplantation (BMT). Further intensive chemotherapy is indicated to re-induce remission in cases that relapse after 1 year of treatment.
- BMT is also indicated in cases with a poor prognosis and in the second and third remission.
- Allogenic BMT has a 5-year relapse-free survival rate of 65% in the second remission and a 3-year survival rate of 55% in the first remission. Leukaemia cells are destroyed by chemotherapy (e.g. cyclophosphamide) plus total body irradiation. Immunosuppressive therapy such as cyclosporin and methotrexate is used to prevent graft versus host disease after allogenic BMT.
- Autologous BMT is also possible, but with less impressive results.
- Treatment of adult ALL is similar to that of childhood ALL. However, the induction and maintenance treatments are more intense in view of the poorer prognosis.
- Supportive care includes blood and platelet transfusions, antimicrobials and allopurinol.
- AML.
  - Induction of remission is achieved with cytosine arabinoside, doxorubicin and 6-thioguanine. The mortality risk during induction is 10%.
  - Maintenance therapy includes cytosine arabinoside, cyclophosphamide, methotrexate, etoposide, 5-azacytidine and 6-mercaptopurine.
  - Arsenic trioxide seems to be promising in the treatment of acute promyelocytic leukaemia (PML). The mechanism of action seems to involve the PML–retinoic acid receptor-alpha (PML-RAR-alpha) fusion protein.
  - All-*trans*-retinoic acid (ATRA) is used in patients with $M_5$ to prevent disseminated intravascular coagulopathy (DIC).
  - Supportive care includes blood and platelet transfusions, IV fluids, IV antimicrobials, haematopoietic growth factors, aseptic techniques when dealing with central venous catheters (e.g. Hickman line) and allopurinol.
  - Relapse is treated by re-induction chemotherapy or BMT.

# Prognosis

- ALL.
  - The overall 5-year survival rate is 80% in girls and 50% in boys. The prognosis is worse in adults.
- AML.
  - The overall 10-year disease-free survival rate is 25%. The prognosis is worse in patients over 30 years of age and with a high WBC.

# 50 Chronic leukaemia

## Epidemiology

- Chronic lymphocytic leukaemia (CLL) is a disease of the elderly.
- Chronic myelocytic leukaemia (CML) occurs in all age groups.

## Aetiology

- *See* aetiology of acute leukaemia on page 144.
- Philadelphia chromosome (reciprocal translocation of part of the long arm of chromosome 22 to chromosome 9) occurs in most cases of CML. In this myeloproliferative disorder the t(9;22) reciprocal translocation results in the generation of a novel fusion oncoprotein, BCR-ABL, with constitutive tyrosine kinase activity.
- Trisomy of chromosome 12 and deletion 13q14 occur in CLL.
- There is p53- and RB1-altered expression.

## Pathology

- Around 95% of CLL cases are of the B-cell type. The T-cell type (5% of cases) causes less immunoglobulin suppression and less lymphadenopathy. Autoimmune haemolytic anaemia occurs in 10% of CLL patients.
- Hypercellular bone marrow with lymphocytic or myeloid replacement.
- Infiltration of liver, spleen and lymph nodes.

- CLL can be subdivided into four stages depending upon the presence of anaemia, lymphadenopathy, splenomegaly and thrombocytopenia.

# Clinical features

- The patient may be asymptomatic.
- Symptoms include malaise, fatigue, weight loss, bruising and bleeding, abdominal discomfort, bone pains and fever.
- Signs include pallor, purpura, lymphadenopathy (especially in CLL), splenomegaly, hepatomegaly and signs of infection.

# Investigations

- Blood count and film. In CLL the lymphocyte count exceeds $10 \times 10^9/l$ (small well-differentiated lymphocytes). In CML there is leukocytosis with an increase in all granulocyte series, especially myelocytes. Anaemia and thrombocytopenia are common.
- Bone-marrow examination.
- Lymph-node biopsy.
- Leukocyte alkaline phosphatase.

# Treatment

- No treatment is indicated in asymptomatic patients. Blood counts are monitored regularly.
- Symptomatic patients with CLL are treated with chlorambucil (3 mg daily) until remission occurs. Relapse is treated with further chemotherapy. Other effective drugs include fludarabine and prednisolone. The latter is particularly useful in patients with bone-marrow failure.
- Symptomatic patients with CML are treated with busulfan (70 mg/kg) until remission occurs (WBC $< 20 \times 10^9/l$). Relapse is treated with further chemotherapy. Other effective drugs include hydroxyurea and interferon-$\alpha$.

- Imatinib mesylate represents the first of a new generation of molecular-targeted therapies for chronic myeloid leukaemia. This agent inhibits the tyrosine kinase activity of BCR-ABL.
- Blastic transformation of CML is treated appropriately as for AML and ALL.
- Allogenic BMT is considered during the first remission in patients with CML who are under 50 years of age and have a matched donor.
- Supportive care includes treatment of infections and transfusion of blood products (platelets and red blood cells).

# Prognosis

- CLL.
  - The overall median survival is 5 years.
  - Poor prognostic indicators include lymphadenopathy, splenomegaly, anaemia and thrombocytopenia.
- CML.
  - The 5-year survival rate is less than 5%.
  - Allogenic BMT in suitable patients appears to cure 40% of patients, but long-term results are still awaited.
  - The Philadelphia-negative type has a poorer prognosis.

# Hairy cell leukaemia

- This is regarded as a B-cell leukaemia.
- It is more common in males, especially during the sixth and seventh decades of life.
- It is usually readily diagnosed by observation of typical hairy cells (HCs) in the blood film. The diagnosis is then confirmed by tartrate-resistant acid phosphatase staining, marker analysis and bone-marrow examination.
- Anaemia, thrombocytopenia, neutropenia and splenomegaly are common features.
- Chlorodeoxyadenosine is the treatment of first choice. Deoxycoformycin and rituximab (anti-CD20) are useful for the treatment of relapsed/refractory disease.

# 51 Hodgkin's lymphoma

## Epidemiology

- The incidence is approximately 1.8 per 100 000 per year in Western countries. However, there is geographical variation.
- The incidence shows a bimodal age distribution with the first peak occurring between the ages of 15 and 30 years and the second peak occurring above the age of 50 years.
- The male:female ratio is 1.5:1.

## Aetiology

- Familial tendency.
- The human leukocyte antigens (HLAs) HLA-A1 and HLA-A12 are both associated with the disease.
- Epstein–Barr virus genome can be detected in 40% of all cases.

## Pathology

- Reed–Sternberg or mononuclear Hodgkin's cells are characteristic.
- Histological types:
  - lymphocyte-depleted
  - lymphocyte-predominant
  - mixed cellularity
  - nodular sclerosis.

- The lymphocyte-predominant type has the best prognosis, whereas the lymphocyte-depleted type carries a poor prognosis.

# Clinical features

- Lymphadenopathy. The neck is the most frequent site at presentation (70% of cases), followed by the axilla (20%) and groin (10%).
- Constitutional symptoms (fever, weight loss, pruritus and sweats) occur in 25% of patients. Alcohol-induced pain is reported in 3% of cases.
- Other features include autoimmune haemolytic anaemia, immune thrombocytopenia, erythema multiforme, erythroderma, lymphoderma, superior/inferior vena cava obstruction, obstructive jaundice, ureteric obstruction and paraneoplastic syndromes.
- Hodgkin's disease may involve the spinal cord, lung, bone marrow, skin, gut, liver and/or spleen.

# Investigations

- FBC, ESR and serum biochemistry.
- CXR (mediastinal and bronchopulmonary lymphadenopathy, thymus enlargement).
- Thoracic and abdominal CT.
- Positron emission tomographic (PET) scanning. As it assesses differences in the metabolic activity of cancer cells, PET scanning may be superior to computerised tomographic scanning, which is limited to showing structural anatomical abnormalities.
- Biopsy (excisional or percutaneous).
- Other investigations include lymphangiography, bone-marrow trephine and bone scan.
- Barium studies (if indicated).

# Ann Arbor staging system

- Stage I: involvement of a single node region or a single extra-lymphatic site or organ.
- Stage II: involvement of two or more node regions on the same side of the diaphragm. Involvement of a single extranodal site plus one (or more) node regions on the same side of the diaphragm.
- Stage III: involvement of lymph nodes on both sides of the diaphragm which may include the spleen or an extranodal site.
- Stage IV: diffuse involvement of one or more extra-lymphatic organs.
- A: no constitutional symptoms.
- B: constitutional symptoms present.

# Treatment

- Standard treatment consists of combined-modality therapy that includes an abbreviated course of chemotherapy and involved-field radiation. As this continues to include radiation therapy, patients will remain at risk of long-term toxicities that include the development of second cancers and cardiovascular events. Recent studies testing the role of chemotherapy alone are now available. They demonstrate that the omission of radiation therapy results in a small but statistically significant reduction in disease control, but no detectable differences in overall survival. Further follow-up will clarify whether chemotherapy alone is the preferred treatment option. At present patients should be informed of the trade-offs involved in choosing between this option and combined-modality therapy.
- Stages IA and IIA: an abbreviated course of chemotherapy followed by radiotherapy to the involved and adjacent lymph nodes (40 Gy in 20 fractions).
- Stage IIIA: combination chemotherapy, such as MOPP (mustine, oncovin, procarbazine and prednisolone) or ABVD (adriamycin, bleomycin, vinblastine and dacarbazine). Radiotherapy is used for residual and recurrent disease.

- Stages IIB, IIIB and IVB: combination chemotherapy.
- High-dose chemotherapy with stem-cell support is indicated for extensive disease that fails to respond to standard chemotherapy regimens.

# Prognosis

- The 10-year survival rates are as follows:
  - 80% for stage IA
  - 77% for stage IIA
  - 72% for stage IIIA
  - 65% for stage IIB
  - 55% for stage IV.

# 52 Non-Hodgkin's lymphoma (NHL)

## Epidemiology

- The incidence increases with age.
- There is a slight male predominance.
- There is geographical variation in incidence and site. Burkitt's lymphoma (of the jaw) is common in Africa. Middle Eastern lymphoma usually affects the intestine.

## Aetiology

- Viruses – human T-cell leukaemia viruses HTLV1 and HTLV2, Epstein–Barr virus (EBV) and the herpes simplex virus HSV-6 have all been implicated.
- Immunosuppression, including congenital syndromes, and AIDS predispose to NHL.
- Coeliac disease predisposes to T-cell lymphoma of the intestine.
- Genetic factors – chromosomal translocation between chromosomes 8 and 14 and C-myc over-expression – may contribute to aetiology.

## Pathology

- B-cell lymphoma (follicular, diffuse, Waldenström's, chronic lymphocytic leukaemia (CLL), Burkitt's lymphoma and heavy-chain disease) accounts for 90% of cases.

- T-cell lymphoma (cutaneous thymic and peripheral-cell lymphoma) accounts for 10% of cases.
- NHL can be classified as low grade, intermediate grade or high grade.
- Immunological classification is helpful.

# Clinical features

- Lymphadenopathy. The neck is the commonest site.
- Hepatosplenomegaly.
- Compression of structures (e.g. veins, ureters, hepatobiliary ducts, etc.) and constitutional symptoms (fever, sweats and weight loss).

# Staging

- This is the same as for Hodgkin's disease.
- Most patients have stage III or stage IV at presentation.

# Investigations

- FBC and film, ESR, serum biochemistry.
- CXR. Thoracic and abdominal CT.
- Biopsy (excisional or percutaneous).
- Other investigations include bone scan, lymphangiography and bone-marrow trephine.
- Barium studies and IVU may be indicated.

# Treatment

- Follicular lymphoma (40% of cases).
  - Stage I and II (small-cell and mixed) disease is treated by radiotherapy to the involved and adjacent lymph nodes.

- Stage I and II (large-cell) disease is treated by radiotherapy and chemotherapy (CHOP regimen: cyclophosphamide, doxorubicin, vincristine and prednisolone).
  - Stage III and IV disease is treated with chemotherapy (low-dose or high-dose) and interferon-α.
- Intermediate- and high-grade lymphoma (diffuse) is treated with combination chemotherapy (high-dose).
- High-dose chemotherapy with peripheral stem-cell support or autologous bone-marrow transplantation is indicated for NHL that is unresponsive to standard regimens, and for recurrent disease.
- Large-cell NHL in childhood is treated with an intensive induction course of chemotherapy followed by a consolidation phase and a maintenance course of alternating pairs of drugs.
- Recent research suggests that rituximab is safe and effective in the treatment of refractory or relapsed low-grade or follicular CD20 B-cell non-Hodgkin's lymphoma.

# Prognosis

- Follicular lymphoma has a 10-year survival rate of:
  - 78% for stage I
  - 60% for stage II
  - 52% for stage III
  - 38% for stage IV.
- Diffuse intermediate and high-grade NHL has a 3-year disease-free survival rate of 50%.
- Large NHL in childhood has a 5-year survival rate of 70% with modern management.
- Recurrent disease has a 3-year survival rate of 35% with high-dose chemotherapy.

# 53 Multiple myeloma

## Epidemiology

- The incidence is approximately 3 per 100 000 per year. It increases with age.
- Men are more commonly affected than women.

## Pathology

- Infiltration of bone and bone marrow by malignant plasma cells causing osteoporosis, osteopenia, lytic lesions and pathological fractures.
- Paraproteinaemia (IgG, IgA, Bence–Jones, IgM and/or IgD) occurs in 99% of cases.
- Renal impairment (light-chain deposition in the distal tubule, hyperuricaemia, amyloidosis and hypercalcaemia).

## Clinical features

- Diffuse bone pain is the commonest symptom (67% of cases). Pathological fractures and cord compression may occur.
- Anaemia, recurrent infections, fatigue, nausea and hypercalcaemia.
- Hyperviscosity syndrome.
- Hepatomegaly, splenomegaly and lymphadenopathy are uncommon.

- Other clinical features include congestive cardiac failure and renal impairment.

# Investigations

- FBC, ESR, serum biochemistry and viscosity.
- Serum immunoglobulins and immunoelectrophoresis.
- $\beta_2$-microglobulin–plasma/urine.
- Bone-marrow aspiration and trephine.
- 24-hour urinary light chains, proteins and calcium.
- Radiological skeletal survey.

# Treatment

- Serious complications (e.g. dehydration, hypercalcaemia and spinal cord compression) should be treated promptly with appropriate measures (e.g. fluid replacement, bisphosphonates and radiotherapy to the spinal cord).
- Combined melphalan–prednisolone oral therapy is the first line of treatment (6 to 9 courses). $H_2$-antagonists are usually added to therapy and interferon-$\alpha$ may be used as a maintenance therapy. The response rate is 60%. Some centres use more complex regimens of combination chemotherapy.
- Second-line chemotherapy includes agents such as doxorubicin, vincristine and nitrosoureas. Hemi-body irradiation is also effective as a second-line therapy.
- High-dose chemotherapy and bone-marrow transplantation (autologous or allogenic) may improve outcome in selected patients.
- Radiotherapy for painful bony deposits, spinal cord compression and bones at risk of fracture.
- Internal fixation for pathological fractures and bones at risk.
- Supportive measures (e.g. blood transfusions and antibiotics).
- Monoclonal immunoglobulin levels can be used to monitor response to treatment.
- Recent research suggests that thalidomide has a role to play in the management of multiple myeloma.

# Prognosis

- This depends upon tumour mass.
  - The median survival is 5 years for low tumour mass, 2 years for intermediate tumour mass and 6 months for high tumour mass.
  - High serum urea levels (> 10 mmol/l) and low Hb levels (< 7.5 g/dl) are predictors of poor outcome.

# Waldenström's macroglobulinaemia

- There is production of monoclonal IgM and infiltration of bone marrow by lymphoid cells.
- Clinical features include hyperviscosity, weakness, haemolytic anaemia, purpura, bleeding disorders, hepatosplenomegaly and lymphadenopathy.
- The disease is slowly progressive, and symptomatic cases require treatment in the form of oral chlorambucil or cyclophosphamide (small dose). Plasmapheresis is effective in reducing hyperviscosity.
- Multiple myeloma chemotherapy protocols can be used to treat aggressive disease.
- The median survival is 4 years.

# 54 Miscellaneous

## Carcinoma of the maxillary antrum

- This is usually diagnosed late after it has invaded surrounding structures.
- Unilateral nasal obstruction and bloodstained nasal discharge are early symptoms. The late clinical features include swelling of the cheek, swelling/ulceration of the palate or the bucco-alveolar sulcus, epiphora, proptosis, diplopia, pain and regional lymphadenopathy (submandibular and cervical).
- Systemic metastases are rare.
- Investigations include plain X-rays, CT and biopsy.
- The tumour is treated by wide local excision (maxillectomy) combined with orbital extenteration if the orbit is involved, followed by radiotherapy.
- Unresectable tumours are treated by radiotherapy and chemotherapy.
- Management also includes reconstruction of surgical defects using temporalis muscle slings, skin grafts or composite bone flaps.
- The 5-year survival rate is 30%.

## Cancer of the nasopharynx

- This type of cancer is relatively common in south China.
- Squamous-cell carcinoma accounts for most cases. Lymphoma and adenoid cystic carcinoma are rare.
- The clinical features include nasal obstruction, bloodstained nasal discharge, cranial nerve palsies and cervical lymphadenopathy.

- Radiotherapy is the mainstay of treatment after three-dimensional radiation planning (up to 15 fields in a single patient). The neck is included in the radiation fields.
- Surgery is reserved for residual or recurrent disease.
- Chemotherapy is used for advanced disease in selected patients.
- The local control rate for T1 and T2 tumours is 90%, compared with 45–75% for T3 and T4 tumours.

# Mesothelioma

- This is a malignant tumour of the pleura or pericardium.
- Pleural mesothelioma is strongly associated with exposure to blue (crocidolite) and brown (amosite) asbestos. The latent interval between exposure and development of disease is approximately 30 years.
- The tumour tends to spread over the pleural surface encasing the lung and to invade the mediastinum, diaphragm and chest wall. A bloodstained pleural effusion is a common finding.
- Patients (aged approximately 60 years) usually present with dyspnoea, cough and chest pain.
- Investigations include CXR, CT, cytological analysis of pleural effusions, thoracoscopy and biopsy.
- Treatment is unsatisfactory. It includes surgical resection for localised lesions, radiotherapy and/or chemotherapy (systemic and/or intrapleural). Cisplatin and interferon-$\alpha$ have a 20% response rate.
- The prognosis is poor, with a median survival of 18 months from diagnosis.

# Chondrosarcoma

- This is the second commonest malignant tumour of bone. The pelvis is most commonly involved.
- The peak incidence occurs in the age range 40–60 years.
- The disease may arise in benign enchondroma.

- Plain X-rays may show bone destruction and flecks of calcification. CT can demonstrate the extent of the lesion.
- Surgical excision of the lesion with endoprosthesis (if required) is the mainstay of management.
- Radiotherapy is used for palliation. Chemotherapy is occasionally used.

# Ewing's sarcoma

- This is a malignant round-cell tumour of bone with a peak incidence during the second decade of life.
- The pelvis and femur are most commonly affected.
- Clinical features include swelling, pain, fever, weight loss and dyspnoea due to pulmonary metastases.
- Investigations include plain X-rays, CT, MRI and biopsy.
- Treatment consists of radical radiotherapy combined with adjuvant chemotherapy (doxorubicin, cyclophosphamide, vincristine, actinomycin D and ifosfamide).
- The 5-year survival rate for patients with localised disease is 55%.

# Cutaneous T-cell lymphoma ('mycosis fungoides')

- The peak incidence occurs during the fifth and sixth decades of life.
- It is equally common in men and women.
- The disease has four stages:
  - stage I – plaque or eczematous skin lesions
  - stage II – plaque with enlarged lymph nodes that are pathologically negative
  - stage III – erythroderma
  - stage IV – visceral enlargement of pathologically positive nodes.
- Sézary's syndrome is a form of disseminated disease.

- Treatment modalities include PUVA, wide-field radiation, whole-body electron therapy and/or chemotherapy (alkylating agents and interferon).

# Merkel-cell tumour

- This is a rare primary cutaneous neuroendocrine tumour.
- It usually presents as a discrete nodular mass.
- The tumour is primarily treated by surgery and post-operative radiotherapy.
- Chemoradiation is indicated for advanced and recurrent cases.

# Uveal melanoma

- The incidence is 0.6 per 100 000 per year. It is the commonest intra-ocular malignancy in adults.
- Around 85% of lesions arise in the choroidal part, and the remainder arise in the ciliary body and iris.
- Clinical features include a visual field defect, pain, secondary glaucoma and retinal detachment. Systemic metastases are common.
- Treatment modalities include photocoagulation, cryotherapy, radiotherapy and/or surgery.
- Indications for enucleation include pain, secondary glaucoma, invasion of surrounding structures and macular/optic nerve involvement.

# Squamous-cell carcinoma of the bladder

- This accounts for 3% of all bladder cancers.
- Risk factors include:
  - chronic infection (e.g. *Schistosoma haematobium* cystitis)
  - stones
  - long-term catheterisation and neuropathic bladders.

- The disease is usually advanced at presentation.
- The tumour is treated by radical cystectomy.
- The tumour is not radiosensitive.

# Neuroblastoma

- This arises from adrenal or neural-crest tissue.
- It occurs in 1 in 10 000 live births.
- Clinical features include abdominal mass, neurological signs and symptoms, Horner's syndrome and distant metastases (liver, skin and bone).
- Investigations include bone-marrow aspiration, urinary analysis, VMA, CXR, FBC, serum biochemistry, bone scan, USS, CT and/or MRI.
- Treatment consists of surgical debulking and adjuvant radiotherapy. Other treatment modalities include chemotherapy and autologous bone-marrow transplantation.
- The prognosis depends upon stage, age, location, site of metastases, presentation and the presence of the N-myc oncogene.
- The overall survival rate ranges from 10% to 90% depending upon the stage of the disease.

# 55 Long-term venous access

## Indications

- Administration of cytotoxic drugs.
- Total parenteral nutrition (TPN).
- Transfusion of blood products.
- Administration of antimicrobials.
- Bone-marrow or peripheral stem-cell infusion.

## Catheters

- These are usually made of silicone (which has low thrombogenicity and is flexible) or polyurethane.
- They can be single, double or triple lumen. The latter type is associated with a higher incidence of sepsis.
- Hickman lines are wide-bore silicone catheters which were first described in 1979. Groshing lines are similar to Hickman lines but have self-sealing valves to prevent reflux of blood into the line.

## Insertion techniques

- Catheters can be inserted using a surgical cut-down technique or a percutaneous (Seldinger) introducer kit.
- Ultrasound imaging can be used to guide the procedure.
- The procedure can be performed under general or local anaesthesia.

- The internal jugular, subclavian, external jugular and cephalic veins are usually selected for cannulation. The inferior vena cava is occasionally selected (e.g. in cases of superior vena cava (SVC) obstruction).
- The operating table is tilted head-down to allow distension of veins and prevent air embolism.
- The catheter tip should lie at the right atrium/SVC junction or in the SVC. X-ray control is used to confirm the catheter position.
- The catheter should be tunnelled subcutaneously so that the exit point is approximately 15 cm down the chest wall. Tunnelling aids line stabilisation and reduces the infection risk.
- A Dacron cuff is positioned near the skin exit site, and the induced fibrosis aids stabilisation of the line.
- Totally implantable devices have ports or reservoirs with a self-sealing silicone septum (e.g. Port-Cath).
- Totally implantable pumps are also available.

# Complications

- Sepsis.
  - Skin exit site infection requires dressing and antimicrobials (e.g. vancomycin).
  - Tunnel infection requires catheter removal.
  - Catheter tip infection responds to vancomycin if it is due to *Staphylococcus epidermidis*. Removal is frequently required.
- The incidence of pneumothorax should be less than 3%.
- Air embolism.
- Injury of neighbouring structures during catheter insertion.
- Catheter fracture.
- Catheter occlusion can be treated with heparin or streptokinase (250 000 units). Low-dose warfarin can be used to prevent obstruction due to clot formation.
- Vein thrombosis.
- Extravasation of drugs can occur with totally implantable devices.

# Principles of catheter care

- Aseptic technique.
- Flushing with heparin/saline once weekly if the catheter is not in regular use. Totally implantable devices may be flushed once monthly.
- Nurses' training.
- Patients' education.

# 56 Pain control in advanced cancer

- Pain is a complex symptom with sensory and emotional components. Its severity should be decided by the patient and not by the carer.
- Empathy, good communication skills and regular assessment are essential to pain management.
- The cause of pain should be accurately diagnosed and removed if possible.
- The analgesic is chosen in a stepped approach (the analgesic ladder) as follows.
  - Step 1: non-opioids (e.g. paracetamol 1 g 6-hourly, ibuprofen 200–600 mg 8-hourly, diclofenac 50 mg 8-hourly, Entonox, nefopam, etc.).
  - Step 2: weak opioids (e.g. codeine and dihydrocodeine).
  - Step 3: strong opioids (e.g. morphine, diamorphine for subcutaneous route and fentanyl for transdermal administration).
- The starting dose of strong opioids depends upon the previous analgesic needs and on renal function. Hepatic dysfunction has a limited clinical impact on opiate metabolism.
- Secondary analgesia relieves pain through an indirect mechanism. Secondary analgesics include antidepressants (e.g. amitriptyline, lofepramine), corticosteroids, antispasmodics (e.g. hyoscine butylbromide), carbamazepine, sodium valproate and membrane-stabilising drugs.
- Spinal analgesia via an intrathecal catheter (strong opioid/bupivacaine mixture) has a role in patients who are unable to tolerate the adverse effects of systemic opioids.
- Peripheral nerve blocks may also be used in pain control.
- The management of bone metastases also includes radiotherapy, orthopaedic fixation of pathological fractures, bisphosphonates

(e.g. clodronate), nerve block and hormonal manipulation where appropriate.

- Neurosurgical procedures for pain control (e.g. cordotomy for unilateral pain) are occasionally required, and liaison with neurosurgical colleagues is needed.

# 57 Symptom control in advanced cancer

- Pain is a complex symptom with sensory and emotional components. Its severity should be decided by the patient and not by the carer (*see* Chapter 56).
- Nausea and vomiting.
  - The choice of an anti-emetic depends upon the cause. A single anti-emetic is sufficient in most cases.
  - The cause (e.g. hypercalcaemia) should be specifically treated if appropriate.
  - Antihistamines such as cyclizine and hyoscine hydrobromide are effective in the treatment of vomiting due to stimulation of vomiting centres.
  - Potent dopamine antagonists such as haloperidol are effective in the treatment of vomiting due to stimulation of the chemoreceptor trigger zone.
  - Peripheral dopamine antagonists such as metoclopramide and domperidone are effective in the treatment of vomiting due to gastric stasis.
  - Other useful anti-emetics include ondansetron (serotonin antagonist) and cisapride (gastrointestinal stimulant).
  - Associated management of nausea and vomiting includes dexamethasone, nasogastric drainage and percutaneous gastrostomy.
- Dysphagia.
  - Malignant dysphagia can be relieved by oesophageal intubation, radiotherapy, laser therapy or dexamethasone.
  - Viral infections and candidiasis causing dysphagia should be appropriately treated (e.g. with fluconazole, Zovirax, etc.).

- Hydration and feeding can be achieved via gastrostomy.
- The swallowing therapist may play an important role.
- Bowel obstruction.
  - The causes include recurrent abdominal tumour, metastatic obstruction, a primary tumour, constipation, benign adhesions and ileus.
  - Surgery should be considered in fit patients with obstruction that is suspected to be due to a single site obstruction or benign adhesions, provided that the patient is willing to undergo surgery.
  - Hyoscine can be used to relieve colic.
  - Most patients will absorb sufficient fluid from their upper GI tract to prevent symptomatic dehydration. Parenteral nutrition is only indicated during pre-operative preparation for surgery.
- Diarrhoea.
  - Causes such as constipation, infection, partial bowel obstruction, carcinoid syndrome and post-gastrectomy syndrome should be considered.
  - Management includes rehydration and loperamide.
  - Management of steatorrhoea includes loperamide, ranitidine, pancreatin supplement and/or biliary drainage (bypass surgery or endoscopic stenting).
  - Blind-loop syndrome can be treated with antibiotics (e.g. tetracycline, metronidazole).
  - Radiotherapy-induced diarrhoea responds to non-steroidal anti-inflammatory drugs (NSAIDs).
  - Octreotide is used to treat severe refractory diarrhoea.
- Constipation.
  - This should be prevented in high-risk patients by regular use of co-danthrusate (2 capsules at night). The laxative dose is titrated according to the opiate dose in order to maintain comfortable stools.
  - If the rectum is full, constipation is treated with glycerine suppositories and phosphate enemas. If this approach is unsuccessful, manual evacuation under sedation should be considered.
  - Other drugs used in the treatment of constipation include bisacodyl (10–20 mg orally or by rectum) and docusate (100–300 mg three times a day).

- Oral problems.
  - Oral hygiene is essential.
  - Aphthous ulceration is treated with tetracycline suspension and topical corticosteroids.
  - Fungal infections are treated with fluconazole (a single dose) and nystatin suspension.
  - Benzydamine hydrochloride (Difflam) mouthwash provides effective oral analgesia.
- Anorexia.
  - This can be helped with corticosteroids (e.g. dexamethasone 4 mg daily) or megestrol (160 mg daily).
- Ascites.
  - The commonest causes of malignant ascites are carcinomas of the bronchus, breast, stomach, pancreas, colon and ovary.
  - Paracentesis offers immediate relief, and can be achieved using a peritoneal dialysis catheter inserted through the left iliac fossa or the mid-line suprapubically under local anaesthesia. The ascites is drained to dryness over a period of 6 hours and a colostomy bag is placed over the puncture site.
  - Spironolactone combined with frusemide aids long-term control.
  - A peritoneo-venous shunt (LeVeen shunt) can be inserted under a general anaesthetic in suitable patients.
- Pleural effusions.
  - Pleural effusions are worth draining (1.5 l at a time) if they are symptomatic. If the effusion recurs, pleurodesis with 1 g of tetracycline is indicated after drainage to dryness through an intercostal drain. Talc powder achieves 100% control rate but causes a vigorous reaction.
  - Pleuroperitoneal shunt is a recognised treatment modality in selected patients.
- Anxiety and depression.
  - Anxiety is relieved by empathy, explanation, counselling and relaxation.
  - Depression (early-morning wakening, self-blame, feelings of worthlessness and loss of interest in life) can be effectively treated with antidepressants (e.g. amitriptyline 75–150 mg daily or lofepramine 140–210 mg daily).

# Index